*Principles of Adolescent
Substance Use Disorder Treatment:
A Research-Based Guide*

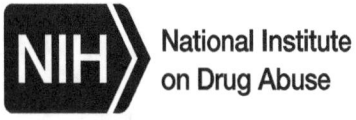

***Principles of Adolescent
Substance Use Disorder Treatment:
A Research-Based Guide***

This publication is in the public domain and may be used or reproduced in
its entirety without permission from NIDA. Citation of the source is appreciated.

NIDA wishes to thank the following individuals for their helpful comments during the review of this publication:

Tina Burrell, M.A., Washington State Department of Social and Health Services

Connie Cahalan, Missouri Department of Mental Health

Barbara Cimaglio, Vermont Department of Health

Michael L. Dennis, Ph.D., Chestnut Health Systems

Rochelle Head-Dunham, M.D., Louisiana Department of Health and Hospitals

Scott W. Henggeler, Ph.D., Medical University of South Carolina

Sharon Levy, M.D., M.P.H., Children's Hospital Boston

Kenneth J. Martz, Psy.D., CAS, Pennsylvania Department of Drug and Alcohol Programs

Kathy Paxton, M.S., West Virginia Bureau for Behavioral Health and Health Facilities

Paula D. Riggs, M.D., University of Colorado School of Medicine

Contents

FROM THE DIRECTOR 1

I. INTRODUCTION 2

II. PRINCIPLES OF ADOLESCENT SUBSTANCE USE DISORDER TREATMENT 8
   1. Adolescent substance use needs to be identified and addressed as soon as possible 9
   2. Adolescents can benefit from a drug abuse intervention even if they are not addicted to a drug 9
   3. Routine annual medical visits are an opportunity to ask adolescents about drug use 9
   4. Legal interventions and sanctions or family pressure may play an important role in getting adolescents to enter, stay in, and complete treatment 9
   5. Substance use disorder treatment should be tailored to the unique needs of the adolescent 9
   6. Treatment should address the needs of the whole person, rather than just focusing on his or her drug use 10
   7. Behavioral therapies are effective in addressing adolescent drug use 10
   8. Families and the community are important aspects of treatment 10
   9. Effectively treating substance use disorders in adolescents requires also identifying and treating any other mental health conditions they may have 10
   10. Sensitive issues such as violence and child abuse or risk of suicide should be identified and addressed 11
   11. It is important to monitor drug use during treatment 11
   12. Staying in treatment for an adequate period of time and continuity of care afterward are important 11
   13. Testing adolescents for sexually transmitted diseases like HIV, as well as hepatitis B and C, is an important part of drug treatment 11

III. FREQUENTLY ASKED QUESTIONS 12
   1. Why do adolescents take drugs? 13
   2. What drugs are most frequently used by adolescents? 13
   3. How do adolescents become addicted to drugs, and which factors increase risk? 14
   4. Is it possible for teens to become addicted to marijuana? 14
   5. Is abuse of prescription medications as dangerous as other forms of illegal drug use? 15
   6. Are steroids addictive and can steroid abuse be treated? 15
   7. How do other mental health conditions relate to substance use in adolescents? 16
   8. Does treatment of ADHD with stimulant medications like Ritalin® and Adderall® increase risk of substance abuse later in life? 16
   9. What are signs of drug use in adolescents, and what role can parents play in getting treatment? 16
   10. How can parents participate in their adolescent child's treatment? 17
   11. What role can medical professionals play in addressing substance abuse (including abuse of prescription drugs) among adolescents? 17
   12. Is adolescent tobacco use treated similarly to other drug use? 18
   13. Are there medications to treat adolescent substance abuse? 18
   14. Do girls and boys have different treatment needs? 18
   15. What are the unique treatment needs of adolescents from different racial/ethnic backgrounds? 19
   16. What role can the juvenile justice system play in addressing adolescent drug abuse? 19
   17. What role do 12-step groups or other recovery support services play in addiction treatment for adolescents? 19

IV. TREATMENT SETTINGS	20
Outpatient/Intensive Outpatient	21
Partial Hospitalization	21
Residential/Inpatient Treatment	21
V. EVIDENCE-BASED APPROACHES TO TREATING ADOLESCENT SUBSTANCE USE DISORDERS	22
BEHAVIORAL APPROACHES	23
Adolescent Community Reinforcement Approach (A-CRA)	23
Cognitive-Behavioral Therapy (CBT)	24
Contingency Management (CM)	24
Motivational Enhancement Therapy (MET)	24
Twelve-Step Facilitation Therapy	24
FAMILY-BASED APPROACHES	25
Brief Strategic Family Therapy (BSFT)	25
Family Behavior Therapy (FBT)	25
Functional Family Therapy (FFT)	26
Multidimensional Family Therapy (MDFT)	26
Multisystemic Therapy (MST)	26
ADDICTION MEDICATIONS	26
Opioid Use Disorders	27
Alcohol Use Disorders	27
Nicotine Use Disorders	28
RECOVERY SUPPORT SERVICES	28
Assertive Continuing Care (ACC)	28
Mutual Help Groups	29
Peer Recovery Support Services	29
Recovery High Schools	29
TREATMENT REFERRAL RESOURCES	31
REFERENCES	32

From the Director

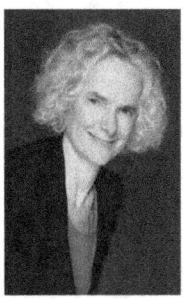

Since its first edition in 1999, NIDA's *Principles of Drug Addiction Treatment* has been a widely used resource for health care providers, families, and others needing information on addiction and treatment for people of all ages. But recent research has greatly advanced our understanding of the particular treatment needs of adolescents, which are often different from those of adults. I thus am very pleased to present this new guide, *Principles of Adolescent Substance Use Disorder Treatment*, focused exclusively on the unique realities of adolescent substance use—which includes abuse of illicit and prescription drugs, alcohol, and tobacco—and the special treatment needs for people aged 12 to 17.

The adolescent years are a key window for both substance use and the development of substance use disorders. Brain systems governing emotion and reward-seeking are fully developed by this time, but circuits governing judgment and self-inhibition are still maturing, causing teenagers to act on impulse, seek new sensations, and be easily swayed by their peers—all of which may draw them to take risks such as trying drugs of abuse. What is more, because critical neural circuits are still actively forming, teens' brains are particularly susceptible to being modified by those substances in a lasting way—making the development of a substance use disorder much more likely.

Addiction is not the only danger. Abusing drugs during adolescence can interfere with meeting crucial social and developmental milestones and also compromise cognitive development. For example, heavy marijuana use in the teen years may cause a loss of several IQ points that are not regained even if users later quit in adulthood. Unfortunately, that drug's popularity among teens is growing—possibly due in part to legalization advocates touting marijuana as a "safe" drug. Nor do most young people appreciate the grave safety risks posed by abuse of other substances like prescription opioids and stimulants or newly popular synthetic cannabinoids ("Spice")—and even scientists still do not know much about how abusing these drugs may affect the developing brain.

These unknowns only add to the urgency of identifying and intervening in substance use as early as possible. Unfortunately, this urgency is matched by the difficulty of reaching adolescents who need help. Only 10 percent of adolescents who need treatment for a substance use disorder actually get treatment. Most teens with drug problems don't want or think they need help, and parents are frequently blind to indications their teenage kids may be using drugs—or they may dismiss drug use as just a normal part of growing up.

Historically the focus with adolescents has tended to be on steering young people clear of drugs before problems arise. But the reality is that different interventions are needed for adolescents at different places along the substance use spectrum, and some require treatment, not just prevention. Fortunately, scientific research has now established the efficacy of a number of treatment approaches that can address substance use during the teen years. This guide describes those approaches, as well as presents a set of guiding principles and frequently asked questions about substance abuse and treatment in this age group. I hope this guide will be of great use to parents, health care providers, and treatment specialists as they strive to help adolescents with substance use problems get the help they need.

Nora D. Volkow, M.D.
Director
National Institute on Drug Abuse

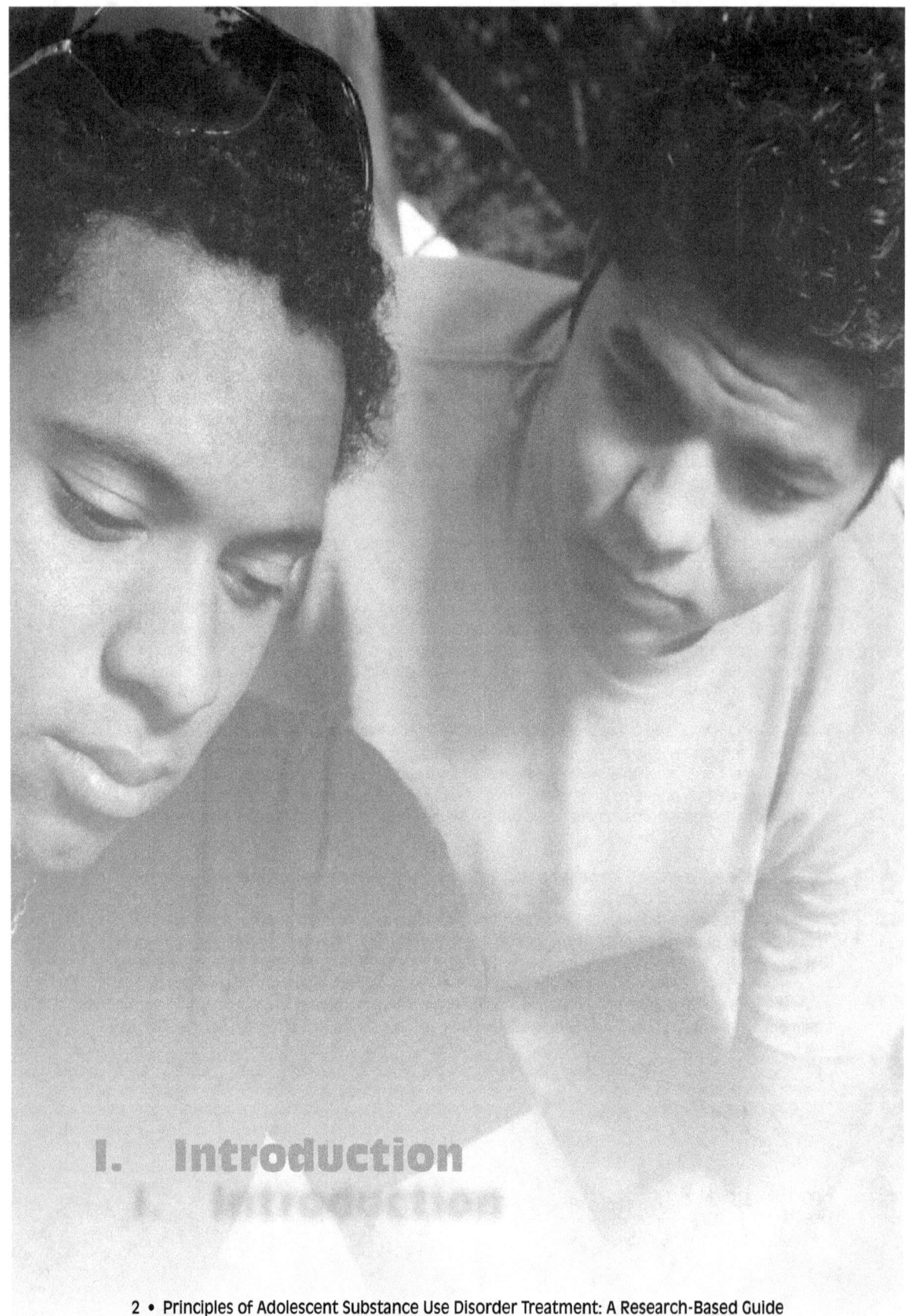

I. Introduction

People are most likely to begin abusing drugs*—including tobacco, alcohol, and illegal and prescription drugs—during adolescence and young adulthood.‡ By the time they are seniors, almost 70 percent of high school students will have tried alcohol, half will have taken an illegal drug, nearly 40 percent will have smoked a cigarette, and more than 20 percent will have used a prescription drug for a nonmedical purpose.[1] There are many reasons adolescents use these substances, including the desire for new experiences, an attempt to deal with problems or perform better in school, and simple peer pressure. Adolescents are "biologically wired" to seek new experiences and take risks, as well as to carve out their own identity. Trying drugs may fulfill all of these normal developmental drives, but in an unhealthy way that can have very serious long-term consequences.

Many factors influence whether an adolescent tries drugs, including the availability of drugs within the neighborhood, community, and school and whether the adolescent's friends are using them. The family environment is also important: Violence, physical or emotional abuse, mental illness, or drug use in the household increase the likelihood an adolescent will use drugs. Finally, an adolescent's inherited genetic vulnerability; personality traits like poor impulse control or a high need for excitement; mental

> The adolescent brain is often likened to a car with a fully functioning gas pedal (the reward system) but weak brakes (the prefrontal cortex).

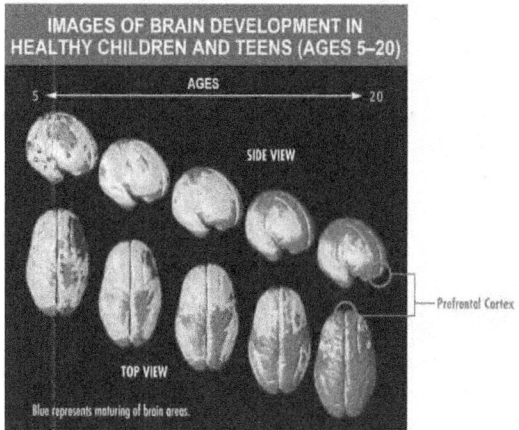

The brain continues to develop through early adulthood. Mature brain regions at each developmental stage are indicated in blue. The prefrontal cortex (red circles), which governs judgment and self-control, is the last part of the brain to mature.
Source: PNAS 101:8174–8179, 2004.

health conditions such as depression, anxiety, or ADHD; and beliefs such as that drugs are "cool" or harmless make it more likely that an adolescent will use drugs.[2]

The teenage years are a critical window of vulnerability to substance use disorders, because the brain is still developing and malleable (a property known as neuroplasticity), and some brain areas are less mature than others. The parts of the brain that process feelings of reward and pain—crucial drivers of drug use—are the first to mature during childhood. What remains incompletely developed during the teen years are the prefrontal cortex and its connections to other brain regions. The prefrontal cortex is responsible for assessing situations, making sound decisions, and controlling our emotions and impulses; typically this circuitry is not mature until a person is in his or her mid-20s (see figure, above).

The adolescent brain is often likened to a car with a fully functioning gas pedal (the reward system) but weak brakes (the prefrontal cortex). Teenagers are highly motivated to pursue pleasurable rewards and avoid pain,

---

* In this guide, the terms *drugs* and *substances* are used interchangeably to refer to tobacco, alcohol, illegal drugs, and prescription medications used for nonmedical reasons.

‡ Specifying the period of *adolescence* is complicated because it may be defined by different variables, and policymakers and researchers may disagree on the exact age boundaries. For purposes of this guide, adolescents are considered to be people between the ages of 12 and 17.

but their judgment and decision-making skills are still limited. This affects their ability to weigh risks accurately and make sound decisions, including decisions about using drugs. For these reasons, adolescents are a major target for prevention messages promoting healthy, drug-free behavior and giving young people encouragement and skills to avoid the temptations of experimenting with drugs.[3]

Most teens do not escalate from trying drugs to developing an addiction or other substance use disorder;* however, even experimenting with drugs is a problem. Drug use can be part of a pattern of risky behavior including unsafe sex, driving while intoxicated, or other hazardous, unsupervised activities. And in cases when a teen does develop a pattern of repeated use, it can pose serious social and health risks, including:

- school failure
- problems with family and other relationships
- loss of interest in normal healthy activities
- impaired memory
- increased risk of contracting an infectious disease (like HIV or hepatitis C) via risky sexual behavior or sharing contaminated injection equipment
- mental health problems—including substance use disorders of varying severity
- the very real risk of overdose death

How drug use can progress to addiction. Different drugs affect the brain differently, but a common factor is that they all raise the level of the chemical *dopamine* in brain circuits that control reward and pleasure.

The brain is wired to encourage life-sustaining and healthy activities through the release of dopamine. Everyday rewards during adolescence—such as hanging out with friends, listening to music, playing sports,

> Despite popular belief, willpower alone is often insufficient to overcome an addiction. Drug use has compromised the very parts of the brain that make it possible to "say no."

and all the other highly motivating experiences for teenagers—cause the release of this chemical in moderate amounts. This reinforces behaviors that contribute to learning, health, well-being, and the strengthening of social bonds.

Drugs, unfortunately, are able to hijack this process. The "high" produced by drugs represents a flooding of the brain's reward circuits with much more dopamine than natural rewards generate. This creates an especially strong drive to repeat the experience. The immature brain, already struggling with balancing impulse and self-control, is more likely to take drugs again without adequately considering the consequences.[4] If the experience is repeated, the brain reinforces the neural links between pleasure and drug-taking, making the association stronger and stronger. Soon, taking the drug may assume an importance in the adolescent's life out of proportion to other rewards.

The development of addiction is like a vicious cycle: Chronic drug use not only realigns a person's priorities but also may alter key brain areas necessary for judgment and self-control, further reducing the individual's ability to control or stop their drug use. This is why, despite popular belief, willpower alone is often insufficient to overcome an addiction. Drug use has compromised the very parts of the brain that make it possible to "say no."

Not all young people are equally at risk for developing an addiction. Various factors including inherited genetic predispositions and adverse experiences in early life make trying drugs and developing a substance use disorder more likely. Exposure to stress (such as emotional or physical abuse) in childhood primes the brain to be sensitive

---

* For purposes of this guide, the term addiction refers to compulsive drug seeking and use that persists even in the face of devastating consequences; it may be regarded as equivalent to a severe substance use disorder as defined by the Diagnostic and Statistical Manual of Mental Disorders, Fifth Edition (DSM-5, 2013). The spectrum of substance use disorders in the DSM-5 includes the criteria for the DSM-4 diagnostic categories of abuse and dependence.

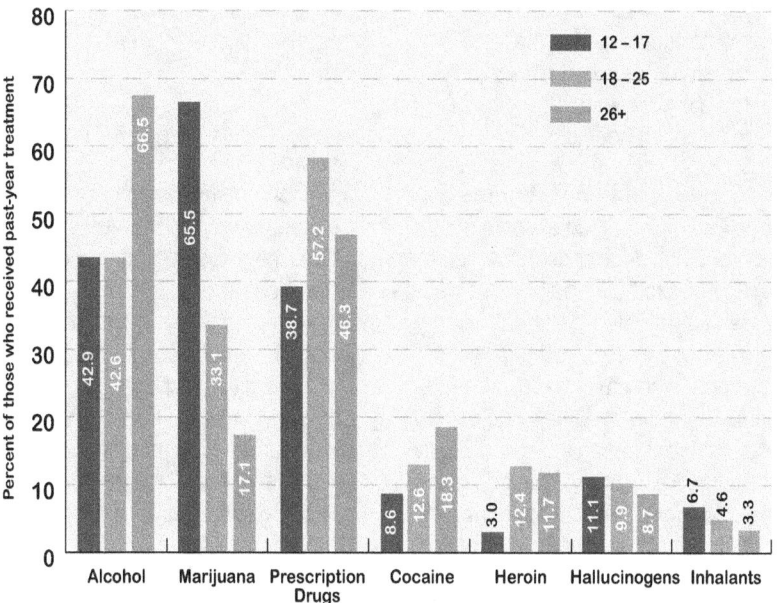

Adolescents Differ from Adults in Substances Most Abused

Source: SAMHSA, Center for Behavioral Health Statistics and Quality, National Survey on Drug Use and Health, 2013.

to stress and seek relief from it throughout life; this greatly increases the likelihood of subsequent drug abuse and of starting drug use early.[5] In fact, certain traits that put a person at risk for drug use, such as being impulsive or aggressive, manifest well before the first episode of drug use and may be addressed by prevention interventions during childhood.[6] By the same token, a range of factors, such as parenting that is nurturing or a healthy school environment, may encourage healthy development and thereby lessen the risk of later drug use.

Drug use at an early age is an important predictor of development of a substance use disorder later. The majority of those who have a substance use disorder started using before age 18 and developed their disorder by age 20.[7] The likelihood of developing a substance use disorder is greatest for those who begin use in their *early* teens. For example, 15.2 percent of people who start drinking by age 14 eventually develop alcohol abuse or dependence (as compared to just 2.1 percent of those who wait until they are 21 or older),[8] and 25 percent of those who begin abusing prescription drugs at age 13 or younger develop a substance use disorder at some time in their lives.[9] Tobacco, alcohol, and marijuana are the first addictive substances most people try. Data collected in 2012 found that nearly 13 percent of those with a substance use disorder began using marijuana by the time they were 14.[10]

When substance use disorders occur in adolescence, they affect key developmental and social transitions, and they can interfere with normal brain maturation. These potentially lifelong consequences make addressing adolescent drug use an urgent matter. Chronic marijuana use in adolescence, for example, has been shown to lead to a loss of IQ that is not recovered even if the individual quits using in adulthood.[11] Impaired memory or thinking ability and other problems caused by drug use can derail a young person's social and educational development and hold him or her back in life.

The serious health risks of drugs compound the need to get an adolescent who is abusing drugs into treatment as quickly as possible. Also, adolescents who are abusing drugs are likely to have other issues such as mental health problems accompanying and possibly contributing to their substance use, and these also need to be addressed.[12] Unfortunately, less than one third of adolescents admitted to substance abuse treatment who have other mental health issues receive any care for their conditions.[13]

Adolescents' drug use and treatment needs differ from those of adults. Adolescents in treatment report abusing different substances than adult patients do. For example, many more people aged 12–17 received treatment for marijuana use than for alcohol use in 2011 (65.5 percent versus 42.9 percent), whereas it was the reverse for adults (see figure, page 5). When adolescents do drink alcohol, they are more likely than adults to binge drink (defined as five or more drinks in a row on a single occasion).[14] Adolescents are less likely than adults to report withdrawal symptoms when not using a drug, being unable to stop using a drug, or continued use of a drug in spite of physical or mental health problems; but they are more likely than adults to report hiding their substance use, getting complaints from others about their substance use, and continuing to use in spite of fights or legal trouble.

Adolescents also may be less likely than adults to feel they need help or to seek treatment on their own. Given their shorter histories of using drugs (as well as parental protection), adolescents may have experienced relatively few adverse consequences from their drug use; their incentive to change or engage in treatment may correspond to the number of such consequences they have experienced.[15] Also, adolescents may have more difficulty than adults seeing their own behavior patterns (including causes and consequences of their actions) with enough detachment to tell they need help.

Only 10 percent of 12- to 17-year-olds needing substance abuse treatment actually receive any services.[16] When they do get treatment, it is often for different reasons than adults. By far, the largest proportion of adolescents who receive treatment are referred by the juvenile justice system (see figure, page 7). Given that adolescents with substance use problems often feel they do not need help, engaging young patients in treatment often requires special skills and patience.

Many treatment approaches are available to address the unique needs of adolescents. The focus of this guide is on *evidence-based* treatment approaches—those that have been scientifically tested and found to be effective in the treatment of adolescent substance abuse. Whether delivered in residential or inpatient settings or offered on an outpatient basis, effective treatments for adolescents primarily consist of some form of behavioral therapy. Addiction medications, while effective and widely prescribed for adults, are not generally approved by the U.S. Food and Drug Administration (FDA) for adolescents. However, preliminary evidence from controlled trials suggest that some medications may assist adolescents in achieving abstinence, so providers may view their young patients' needs on a case-by-case basis in developing a personalized treatment plan.

Whatever a person's age, treatment is not "one size fits all." It requires taking into account the needs of the whole person—including his or her developmental stage and cognitive abilities and the influence of family, friends, and others in the person's life, as well as any additional mental or physical health conditions. Such issues should be addressed at the same time as the substance use treatment. When treating adolescents, clinicians must also be ready and able to manage complications related to their young patients' confidentiality and their dependence on family members who may or may not be supportive of recovery.

Supporting Ongoing Recovery—Sustaining Treatment Gains and Preventing Relapse
Enlisting and engaging the adolescent in treatment is only part of a sometimes long and complex recovery process.[17] Indeed, treatment is often seen as part of a continuum of care. When an adolescent requires substance

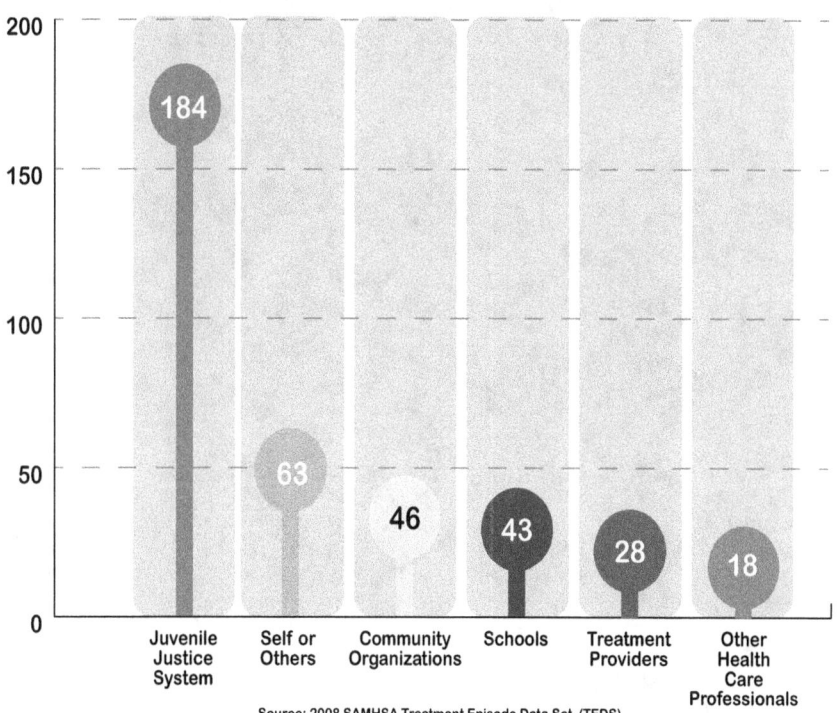

Number of Adolescents Aged 12–17 Admitted to Publicly Funded Substance Abuse Treatment Facilities on an Average Day, by Principal Source of Referral: Treatment Episode Data Set 2008*

Source: 2008 SAMHSA Treatment Episode Data Set (TEDS)

abuse treatment, follow-up care and recovery support (e.g., mutual-help groups like 12-step programs) may be important for helping teens stay off drugs and improving their quality of life.

When substance use disorders are identified and treated in adolescence—especially if they are mild or moderate—they frequently give way to abstinence from drugs with no further problems. Relapse is a possibility, however, as it is with other chronic diseases like diabetes or asthma. Relapse should not be seen as a sign that treatment failed but as an occasion to engage in additional or different treatment. Averting and detecting relapse involves monitoring by the adolescent, parents, and teachers, as well as follow-up by treatment providers. Although recovery support programs are not a substitute for formal evidence-based treatment, they may help some adolescents maintain a positive and productive drug-free lifestyle that promotes meaningful and beneficial relationships and connections to family, peers, and the community both during treatment and after treatment ends. Whatever services or programs are used, an adolescent's path to recovery will be strengthened by support from family members, non-drug-using peers, the school, and others in his or her life.

---

* "Treatment providers" in this chart refers to "alcohol/drug abuse care providers." Treatment providers can and do refer people to treatment if, for example, a person is transferring from one level of treatment to another and the original facility does not provide the level of treatment that the person needs, or if a person changes facilities for some other reason. "Other health care professionals" refers to physicians, psychiatrists, or other licensed health care professionals or general hospitals, psychiatric hospitals, mental health programs, or nursing homes.

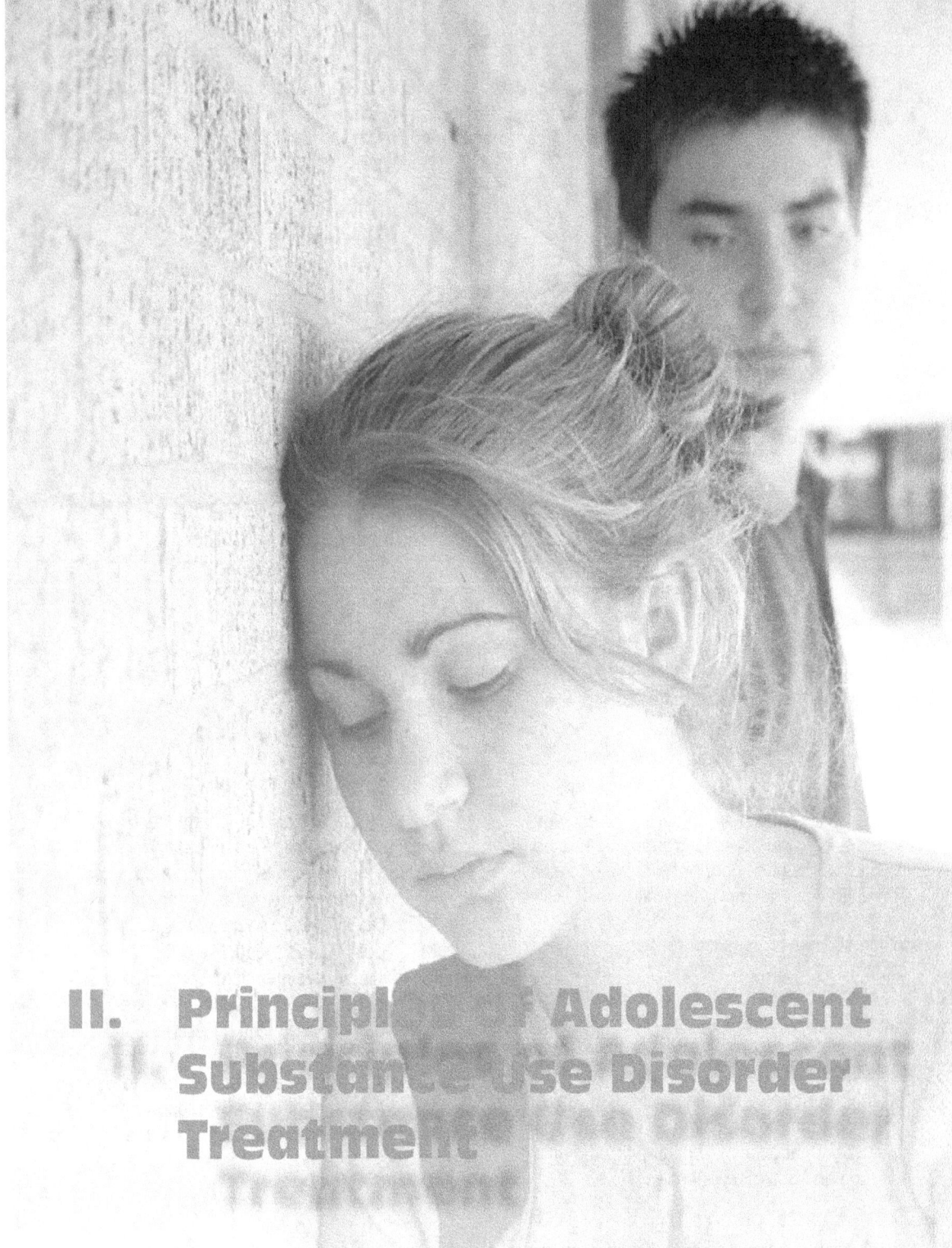

II. Principles of Adolescent Substance Use Disorder Treatment

1. **Adolescent substance use needs to be identified and addressed as soon as possible.** Drugs can have long-lasting effects on the developing brain and may interfere with family, positive peer relationships, and school performance. Most adults who develop a substance use disorder report having started drug use in adolescence or young adulthood, so it is important to identify and intervene in drug use early.

2. **Adolescents can benefit from a drug abuse intervention even if they are not addicted to a drug.**[18] Substance use disorders range from problematic use to addiction and can be treated successfully at any stage, and at any age. For young people, any drug use (even if it seems like only "experimentation"), is cause for concern, as it exposes them to dangers from the drug and associated risky behaviors and may lead to more drug use in the future. Parents and other adults should monitor young people and not underestimate the significance of what may appear as isolated instances of drug taking.

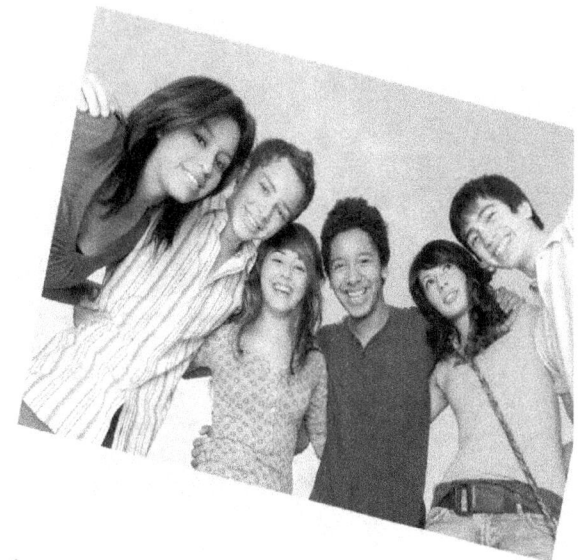

3. **Routine annual medical visits are an opportunity to ask adolescents about drug use.** Standardized screening tools are available to help pediatricians, dentists, emergency room doctors, psychiatrists, and other clinicians determine an adolescent's level of involvement (if any) in tobacco, alcohol, and illicit and nonmedical prescription drug use.[19] When an adolescent reports substance use, the health care provider can assess its severity and either provide an onsite brief intervention or refer the teen to a substance abuse treatment program.[20, 21]

4. **Legal interventions and sanctions or family pressure may play an important role in getting adolescents to enter, stay in, and complete treatment.** Adolescents with substance use disorders rarely feel they need treatment and almost never seek it on their own. Research shows that treatment can work even if it is mandated or entered into unwillingly.[22]

5. **Substance use disorder treatment should be tailored to the unique needs of the adolescent.** Treatment planning begins with a comprehensive assessment to identify the person's strengths and weaknesses to be addressed. Appropriate treatment considers an adolescent's level of psychological development, gender, relations with family and peers, how well he or she is doing in school, the larger community, cultural and ethnic factors, and any special physical or behavioral issues.

Components of Comprehensive Drug Abuse Treatment

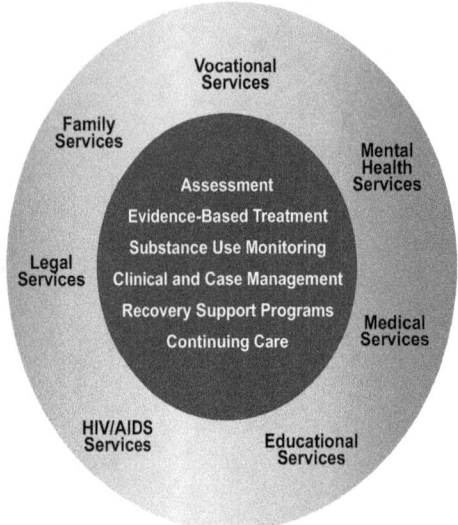

The best treatment programs provide a combination of therapies and other services to meet the needs of the individual patient.

6. **Treatment should address the needs of the whole person, rather than just focusing on his or her drug use.** The best approach to treatment includes supporting the adolescent's larger life needs, such as those related to medical, psychological, and social well-being, as well as housing, school, transportation, and legal services. Failing to address such needs simultaneously could sabotage the adolescent's treatment success.

Many adolescents who abuse drugs have a history of physical, emotional, and/or sexual abuse or other trauma.

7. **Behavioral therapies are effective in addressing adolescent drug use.** Behavioral therapies, delivered by trained clinicians, help an adolescent stay off drugs by strengthening his or her motivation to change. This can be done by providing incentives for abstinence, building skills to resist and refuse substances and deal with triggers or craving, replacing drug use with constructive and rewarding activities, improving problem-solving skills, and facilitating better interpersonal relationships.

8. **Families and the community are important aspects of treatment.** The support of family members is important for an adolescent's recovery. Several evidence-based interventions for adolescent drug abuse seek to strengthen family relationships by improving communication and improving family members' ability to support abstinence from drugs. In addition, members of the community (such as school counselors, parents, peers, and mentors) can encourage young people who need help to get into treatment—and support them along the way.

9. **Effectively treating substance use disorders in adolescents requires also identifying and treating any other mental health conditions they may have.** Adolescents who abuse drugs frequently also suffer from other conditions including depression, anxiety disorders, attention-deficit hyperactivity disorder (ADHD), oppositional defiant disorder, and conduct problems.[23] Adolescents who abuse drugs, particularly those involved in the juvenile justice system, should be screened for other psychiatric disorders. Treatment for these problems should be integrated with the treatment for a substance use disorder.

10. **Sensitive issues such as violence and child abuse or risk of suicide should be identified and addressed.** Many adolescents who abuse drugs have a history of physical, emotional, and/or sexual abuse or other trauma.[24] If abuse is suspected, referrals should be made to social and protective services, following local regulations and reporting requirements.

11. **It is important to monitor drug use during treatment.** Adolescents recovering from substance use disorders may experience relapse, or a return to drug use. Triggers associated with relapse vary and can include mental stress and social situations linked with prior drug use. It is important to identify a return to drug use early before an undetected relapse progresses to more serious consequences. A relapse signals the need for more treatment or a need to adjust the individual's current treatment plan to better meet his or her needs.

12. **Staying in treatment for an adequate period of time and continuity of care afterward are important.** The minimal length of drug treatment depends on the type and extent of the adolescent's problems, but studies show outcomes are better when a person stays in treatment for 3 months or more.[25] Because relapses often occur, more than one episode of treatment may be necessary. Many adolescents also benefit from continuing care following treatment,[26] including drug use monitoring, follow-up visits at home,[27] and linking the family to other needed services.

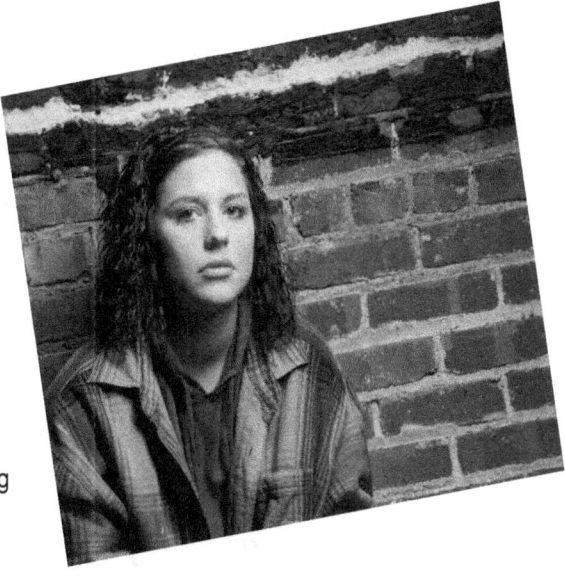

A relapse signals the need for more treatment or a need to adjust the individual's current treatment plan.

13. **Testing adolescents for sexually transmitted diseases like HIV, as well as hepatitis B and C, is an important part of drug treatment.** Adolescents who use drugs—whether injecting or non-injecting—are at an increased risk for diseases that are transmitted sexually as well as through the blood, including HIV and hepatitis B and C. All drugs of abuse alter judgment and decision making, increasing the likelihood that an adolescent will engage in unprotected sex and other high-risk behaviors including sharing contaminated drug injection equipment and unsafe tattooing and body piercing practices—potential routes of virus transmission. Substance use treatment can reduce this risk both by reducing adolescents' drug use (and thus keeping them out of situations in which they are not thinking clearly) and by providing risk-reduction counseling to help them modify or change their high-risk behaviors.[28,29]

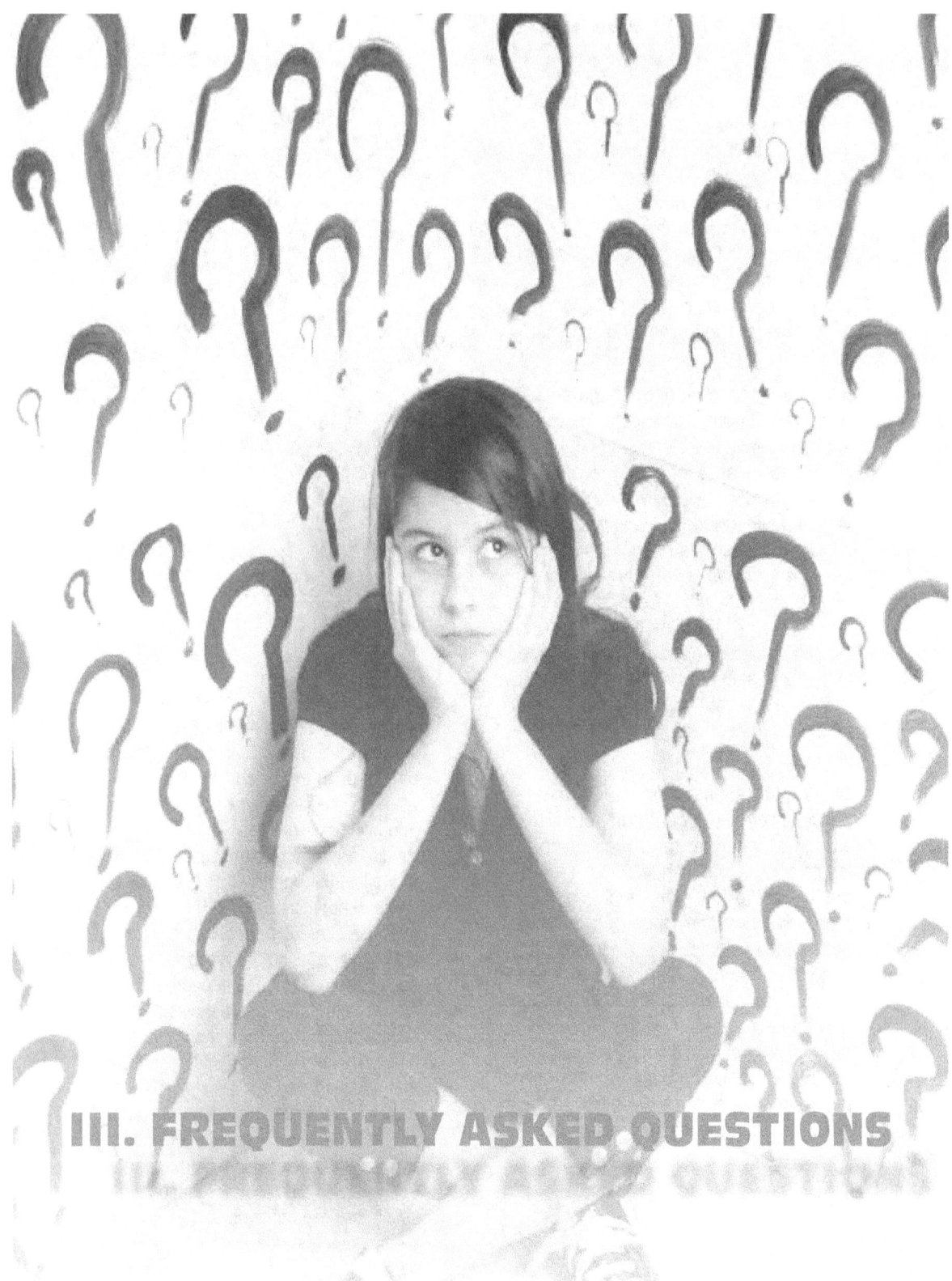

III. FREQUENTLY ASKED QUESTIONS

1. Why do adolescents take drugs?

Adolescents experiment with drugs or continue taking them for several reasons, including:

- **To fit in:** Many teens use drugs "because others are doing it"—or they *think* others are doing it—and they fear not being accepted in a social circle that includes drug-using peers.
- **To feel good:** Abused drugs interact with the neurochemistry of the brain to produce feelings of pleasure. The intensity of this euphoria differs by the type of drug and how it is used.
- **To feel better:** Some adolescents suffer from depression, social anxiety, stress-related disorders, and physical pain. Using drugs may be an attempt to lessen these feelings of distress. Stress especially plays a significant role in starting and continuing drug use as well as returning to drug use (relapsing) for those recovering from an addiction.
- **To do better:** Ours is a very competitive society, in which the pressure to perform athletically and academically can be intense. Some adolescents may turn to certain drugs like illegal or prescription stimulants because they think those substances will enhance or improve their performance.
- **To experiment:** Adolescents are often motivated to seek new experiences, particularly those they perceive as thrilling or daring.

2. What drugs are most frequently used by adolescents?

Alcohol and tobacco are the drugs most commonly abused by adolescents, followed by marijuana. The next most popular substances differ between age groups. Young adolescents tend to favor inhalant substances (such as breathing the fumes of household cleaners, glues, or pens; see "The Dangers of Inhalants," page 15), whereas older teens are more likely to use synthetic marijuana ("K2" or "Spice") and prescription medications—particularly opioid pain relievers like Vicodin® and stimulants like Adderall®. In fact, the Monitoring the Future survey of adolescent drug use and attitudes shows that prescription and over-the-counter medications account for a majority of the drugs most commonly abused by high-school seniors.

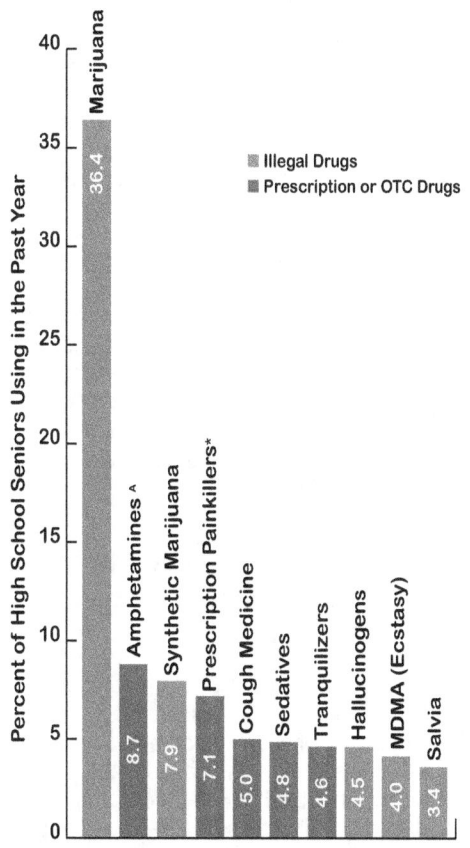

Most Commonly Abused Drugs by High School Seniors (Other than Tobacco and Alcohol)

^The top drug used in this category is Adderall (7.4%)
*The top drugs used in this category are Vicodin (5.3%) and OxyContin (3.6%)
Source: Monitoring the Future National Results on Adolescent Drug Use: Summary of Key Findings, 2013.

3. How do adolescents become addicted to drugs, and which factors increase risk?

Addiction occurs when repeated use of drugs changes how a person's brain functions over time. The transition from voluntary to compulsive drug use reflects changes in the brain's natural inhibition and reward centers that keep a person from exerting control over the impulse to use drugs even when there are negative consequences—the defining characteristic of addiction.

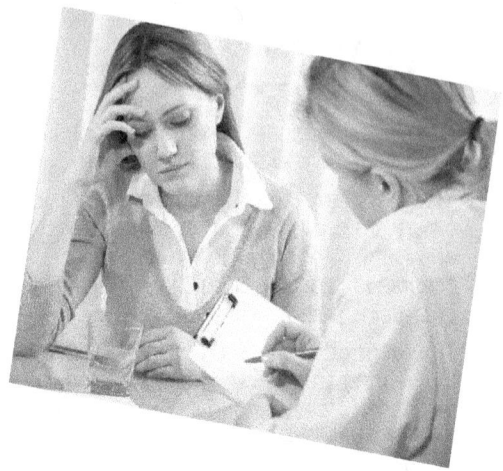

Some people are more vulnerable to this process than others, due to a range of possible risk factors. Stressful early life experiences such as being abused or suffering other forms of trauma are one important risk factor. Adolescents with a history of physical and/or sexual abuse are more likely to be diagnosed with substance use disorders.[30] Many other risk factors, including genetic vulnerability, prenatal exposure to alcohol or other drugs, lack of parental supervision or monitoring, and association with drug-using peers also play an important role.[31]

At the same time, a wide range of genetic and environmental influences that promote strong psychosocial development and resilience may work to balance or counteract risk factors, making it ultimately hard to predict which individuals will develop substance use disorders and which won't.

4. Is it possible for teens to become addicted to marijuana?

Yes. Contrary to common belief, marijuana *is* addictive. Estimates from research suggest that about 9 percent of users become addicted to marijuana; this number increases among those who start young (to about 17 percent, or 1 in 6) and among daily users (to 25–50 percent).[32] Thus, many of the nearly 7 percent of high-school seniors who (according to annual survey data)[33] report smoking marijuana daily or almost daily are well on their way to addiction, if not already addicted, and may be functioning at a sub-optimal level in their schoolwork and in other areas of their lives.

Long-term marijuana users who try to quit report withdrawal symptoms including irritability, sleeplessness, decreased appetite, anxiety, and drug craving, all of which can make it difficult to stay off the drug. Behavioral interventions, including Cognitive-Behavioral Therapy and Contingency Management (providing tangible incentives to patients who remain drug-free) have proven to be effective in treating marijuana addiction (see Page 24 for descriptions of these treatments). Although no medications are currently available to treat marijuana addiction, it is possible that medications to ease marijuana withdrawal, block its intoxicating effects, and prevent relapse may emerge from recent discoveries about the workings of the endocannabinoid system, a signaling system in the body and brain that uses chemicals related to the active ingredients in marijuana.

Legalization of marijuana for adult recreational use and for medicinal purposes is currently the subject of much public debate. Whatever the outcome, public health experts are worried about use increasing among adolescents, since marijuana use as a teen may harm the developing brain, lower IQ, and seriously impair the ability to drive safely, especially when combined with alcohol.

Parents seeking more information about the effects of marijuana on teens are encouraged to see information offered on NIDA's Web site: http://www.drugabuse.gov/drugs-abuse/marijuana.

The Dangers of Inhalants

Various household products, including cleaning fluids, glues, lighter fluid, aerosol sprays, and office supplies like markers and correction fluid, have fumes that are sometimes breathed to obtain a brief, typically alcohol-like high. Because of their ready availability, these are frequently among the earliest substances youth abuse; they are generally less popular among older teens, who have greater access to other substances like alcohol or marijuana.

Although the high from inhalants typically wears off quickly, immediate health consequences of inhalant abuse may be severe: In addition to nausea or vomiting, users risk suffocation and heart failure—called "sudden sniffing death." Serious long-term consequences include liver and kidney damage, hearing loss, bone marrow damage, and brain damage. Although addiction to inhalants is not very common, it can occur with repeated abuse.

Early abuse of inhalants may also be a warning sign for later abuse of other drugs. One study found that youth who used inhalants before age 14 were twice as likely to later use opiate drugs.[34] So it is important for parents to safeguard household products and be alert to signs that their younger teens may be abusing these substances.

5. Is abuse of prescription medications as dangerous as other forms of illegal drug use?

Psychoactive prescription drugs, which include opioid pain relievers, stimulants prescribed for ADHD, and central nervous system depressants prescribed to treat anxiety or sleep disorders, are all effective and safe when taken as prescribed by a doctor for the conditions they are intended to treat. However, they are frequently abused—that is, taken in other ways, in other quantities, or by people for whom they weren't prescribed—and this can have devastating consequences.

In the case of opioid pain relievers such as Vicodin® or OxyContin®, there is a great risk of addiction and death from overdose associated with such abuse. Especially when pills are crushed and injected or snorted, these medications affect the brain and body very much like heroin, including euphoric effects and a hazardous suppression of breathing (the reason for death in cases of fatal opioid overdose). In fact, some young people who develop prescription opioid addictions shift to heroin because it may be cheaper to obtain.[35]

ADHD medications such as Adderall® (which contains the stimulant amphetamine) are increasingly popular among young people who take them believing it will improve their school performance. This too is a dangerous trend. Prescription stimulants act in the brain similarly to cocaine or illegal amphetamines, raising heart rate and blood pressure, as well as producing an addictive euphoria. Other than promoting wakefulness, it is unclear that such medications actually provide much or any cognitive benefit, however, beyond the benefits they provide when taken as prescribed to those with ADHD.[36]

6. Are steroids addictive and can steroid abuse be treated?

Some adolescents—mostly male—abuse anabolic-androgenic steroids in order to improve their athletic performance and/or improve their appearance by helping build muscles. Steroid abuse may lead to serious, even irreversible, health problems including kidney impairment, liver damage, and cardiovascular problems that raise the risk of stroke and heart attack (even in young people). An undetermined percentage of steroid abusers may also become addicted to the drugs—that is, continuing to use them despite physical problems and negative effects on social relations—but the mechanisms causing this addiction are more complex than those for other drugs of abuse.

Steroids are not generally considered intoxicating, but animal studies have shown that chronic steroid use alters the same dopamine reward pathways in the brain that are affected by other substances. Other factors such as underlying body image problems also contribute to steroid abuse.[37] Moreover, when people stop using steroids, they can experience withdrawal symptoms such as hormonal changes that produce fatigue, loss of muscle mass and sex drive, and other unpleasant physical changes. One of the more dangerous withdrawal symptoms is depression, which has led to suicide in some people discontinuing steroids. Steroid abuse is also frequently complicated by abuse of other substances taken either as part of a performance-enhancing regimen (such as stimulants) or to help manage pain-, sleep-, or mood-related side effects (such as opioids, cannabis, and alcohol).[38]

Because of this complicated mix of issues, treatment for steroid abuse necessarily involves addressing all related mental and physical health issues and substance use disorders simultaneously. This may involve behavioral treatments as well as medications to help normalize the hormonal system and treat any depression or pain issues that may be present. If symptoms are severe or prolonged, hospitalization may be needed.

7. How do other mental health conditions relate to substance use in adolescents?

Drug use in adolescents frequently overlaps with other mental health problems. For example, a teen with a substance use disorder is more likely to have a mood, anxiety, learning, or behavioral disorder too. Sometimes drugs can make accurately diagnosing these other problems complicated. Adolescents may begin taking drugs to deal with depression or anxiety, for example; on the other hand, frequent drug use may also cause or precipitate those disorders. Adolescents entering drug abuse treatment should be given a comprehensive mental health screening to determine if other disorders are present. Effectively treating a substance use disorder requires addressing drug abuse and other mental health problems simultaneously.

Addiction occurs when repeated use of drugs changes how a person's brain functions over time.

8. Does treatment of ADHD with stimulant medications like Ritalin® and Adderall® increase risk of substance abuse later in life?

Prescription stimulants are effective at treating attention disorders in children and adolescents, but concerns have been raised that they could make a young person more vulnerable to developing later substance use disorders. On balance, the studies conducted so far have found no differences in later substance use for ADHD-affected children who received treatment versus those that did not. This suggests that treatment with ADHD medication does not affect (either negatively or positively) an individual's risk for developing a substance use disorder.[39]

9. What are signs of drug use in adolescents, and what role can parents play in getting treatment?

If an adolescent starts behaving differently for no apparent reason—such as acting withdrawn, frequently tired or depressed, or hostile–it could be a sign he or she is developing a drug-related problem. Parents and others may overlook such signs, believing them to be a normal part of puberty.

Other signs include:
- a change in peer group
- carelessness with grooming
- decline in academic performance
- missing classes or skipping school
- loss of interest in favorite activities
- changes in eating or sleeping habits
- deteriorating relationships with family members and friends

Parents tend to underestimate the risks or seriousness of drug use. The symptoms listed here suggest a problem that may already have become serious and should be evaluated to determine the underlying cause—which could be a substance abuse problem or another

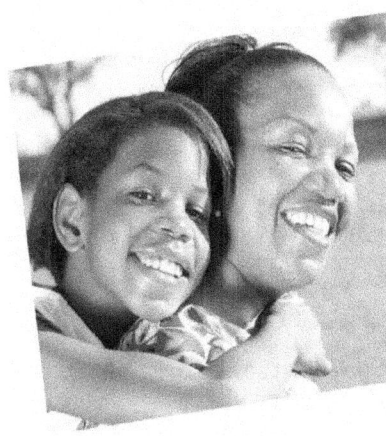

mental health or medical disorder. Parents who are unsure whether their child is abusing drugs can enlist the help of a primary care physician, school guidance counselor, or drug abuse treatment provider.

Parents seeking treatment for an adolescent child are encouraged to see NIDA's booklet, *Seeking Drug Abuse Treatment: Know What to Ask* (http://www.drugabuse.gov/publications/seeking-drug-abuse-treatment) and see the Treatment Referral Resources section of this guide (page 31).

10. How can parents participate in their adolescent child's treatment?

Parents can actively support their child and engage with him or her during the treatment and recovery process. Apart from providing moral and emotional support, parents can also play a crucial role in supporting the practical aspects of treatment, such as scheduling and making appointments, as well as providing needed structure and supervision through household rules and monitoring. Also, several evidence-based treatments for adolescents specifically address drug abuse within the family context. Family-based drug abuse treatment can help improve communication, problem-solving, and conflict resolution within the household. Treatment professionals can help parents and other family members identify ways they can support the changes the adolescent achieves through treatment (see "Family-Based Approaches," pages 25–26).

11. What role can medical professionals play in addressing substance abuse (including abuse of prescription drugs) among adolescents?

Medical professionals have an important role to play in screening their adolescent patients for drug use, providing brief interventions, referring them to substance abuse treatment if necessary, and providing ongoing monitoring and follow-up. Screening and brief interventions do not have to be time-consuming and can be integrated into general medical settings.

- *Screening.* Screening and brief assessment tools administered during annual routine medical checkups can detect drug use before it becomes a serious problem. The purpose of screening is to look for evidence of any use of alcohol, tobacco, or illicit drugs or abuse of prescription drugs and assess how severe the problem is. Results from such screens can indicate whether a more extensive assessment and possible treatment are necessary (see "Screening Tools and Brief Assessments Used with Adolescents," below).[40] Screening as a part of routine care also helps to reduce the stigma associated with being identified as having a drug problem.

Screening Tools and Brief Assessments Used with Adolescents

Screening tools are available and outlined in the American Academy of Pediatrics (AAP) publications, *Tobacco, Alcohol, and Other Drugs: The Role of the Pediatrician in Prevention, Identification, and Management of Substance Abuse*[41] and *Substance Use Screening, Brief Intervention and Referral to Treatment for Pediatricians.*[42]

In addition, the *Alcohol Screening and Brief Intervention for Youth: A Practitioner's Guide* developed by the National Institute on Alcohol Abuse and Alcoholism provides information on identifying adolescents at high risk for alcohol abuse.[43]

- *Brief Intervention.* Adolescents who report using drugs can be given a brief intervention to reduce their drug use and other risky behaviors. Specifically, they should be advised how continued drug use may harm their brains, general health, and other areas of their life, including family relationships and education. Adolescents reporting no substance use can be praised for staying away from drugs and rescreened during their next physical.
- *Referral.* Adolescents with substance use disorders or those that appear to be developing a substance use disorder may need a referral to substance abuse treatment for more extensive assessment and care.
- *Follow-up.* For patients in treatment, medical professionals can offer ongoing support of treatment participation and abstinence from drugs during follow-up visits. Adolescent patients who relapse or show signs of continuing to use drugs may need to be referred back to treatment.
- *Before prescribing medications that can potentially be abused,* clinicians can assess patients for risk factors such as mental illness or a family history of substance abuse, consider an alternative medication with less abuse potential, more closely monitor patients at high risk, reduce the length of time between visits for refills so fewer pills are on hand, and educate both patients and their parents about appropriate use and potential risks of prescription medications, including the dangers of sharing them with others.

12. Is adolescent tobacco use treated similarly to other drug use?

Yes. People often don't think of tobacco use as a kind of "drug abuse" that requires treatment, and motives for quitting smoking may be somewhat different than motives for quitting other drugs. But tobacco use has well-known health risks—especially when begun in the teen years—and the highly addictive nicotine in tobacco can make treatment a necessity to help an adolescent quit. Laboratory research also suggests that nicotine may increase the rewarding and addictive effects of other drugs, making it a potential contributor to other substance use disorders.

Common treatment approaches like Cognitive-Behavioral Therapy are now being used to help adolescents quit smoking (and quit using other drugs) by helping them "train their brains" so they learn to recognize and control their cravings and better deal with life stress. Other therapies like Contingency Management and Motivational Enhancement use incentives and motivation techniques to help teens reduce or stop smoking.[44] (See page 24 for descriptions of these treatments.)

Tobacco use often accompanies other drug use and needs to be addressed as part of other substance use disorder treatment. In a recent survey, nearly 55 percent of current adolescent cigarette smokers (ages 12 to 17) were also illicit drug users (by comparison, only about 6 percent of those who did not smoke used any illicit drugs).[45] Also, cigarette smoking can be an indicator of other psychiatric disorders, which can be identified through comprehensive screening by a treatment provider.

13. Are there medications to treat adolescent substance abuse?

Several medications are approved by the FDA to treat addiction to opioids, alcohol, and nicotine in individuals 18 and older. In most cases, little research has been conducted to evaluate the safety and efficacy of these medications for adolescents; however, some health care providers do use these medications "off-label," especially in older adolescents (see "Addiction Medications," pages 26–28).

14. Do girls and boys have different treatment needs?

Adolescent girls and boys may have different developmental and social issues that may call for different treatment strategies or emphases. For example, girls with substance use disorders may be more likely to also have mood disorders such as depression or to have experienced physical or sexual abuse. Boys with substance use disorders are more likely to also have conduct, behavioral, and learning problems, which may be very disruptive to their school, family, or community. Treatments should take into account the higher rate of internalizing and traumatic stress disorders among adolescent girls, the higher rate of externalizing disruptive disorders and juvenile justice problems among adolescent boys, and other gender differences that may play into adolescent substance use disorders.

15. What are the unique treatment needs of adolescents from different racial/ethnic backgrounds?

Treatment providers are urged to consider the unique social and environmental characteristics that may influence drug abuse and treatment for racial/ethnic minority adolescents, such as stigma, discrimination, and sparse community resources. With the growing number of immigrant children living in the United States, issues of culture of origin, language, and acculturation are important considerations for treatment. The demand for bilingual treatment providers to work with adolescents and their families will also be increasing as the diversity of the U.S. population increases.

16. What role can the juvenile justice system play in addressing adolescent drug abuse?

Involvement in the juvenile justice system is unfortunately a reality for many substance-abusing adolescents, but it presents a valuable opportunity for intervention. Substance use treatment can be incorporated into the juvenile justice system in several ways. These include:
- screening and assessment for drug abuse upon arrest
- initiation of treatment while awaiting trial
- access to treatment programs in the community in lieu of incarceration (e.g., juvenile treatment drug courts)[46,47]
- treatment during incarceration followed by community-based treatment after release

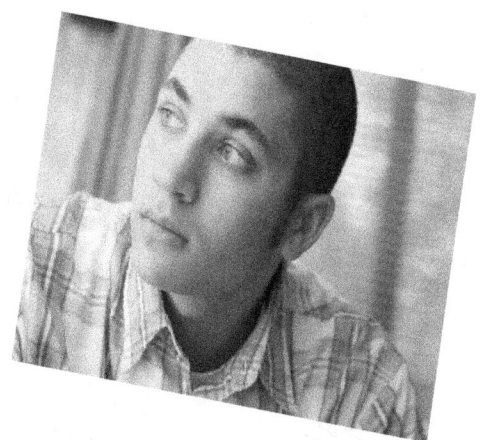

Coordination and collaboration between juvenile justice professionals, drug abuse treatment providers, and other social service agencies are essential in getting needed treatment to adolescent offenders, about one half of whom have substance use disorders.[48]

17. What role do 12-step groups or other recovery support services play in addiction treatment for adolescents?

Adolescents may benefit from participation in self- or mutual-help groups like 12-step programs or other recovery support services, which can reinforce abstinence from drug use and other changes made during treatment, as well as support progress made toward important goals like succeeding in school and reuniting with family. Peer recovery support services and recovery high schools provide a community setting where fellow recovering adolescents can share their experiences and support each other in living a drug-free life.

It is important to note that recovery support services are not a substitute for drug abuse treatment. Also, there is sometimes a risk in support-group settings that conversation among adolescents can turn to talk extolling drug use; group leaders need to be aware of such a possibility and be ready to direct the discussion in more positive directions if necessary.

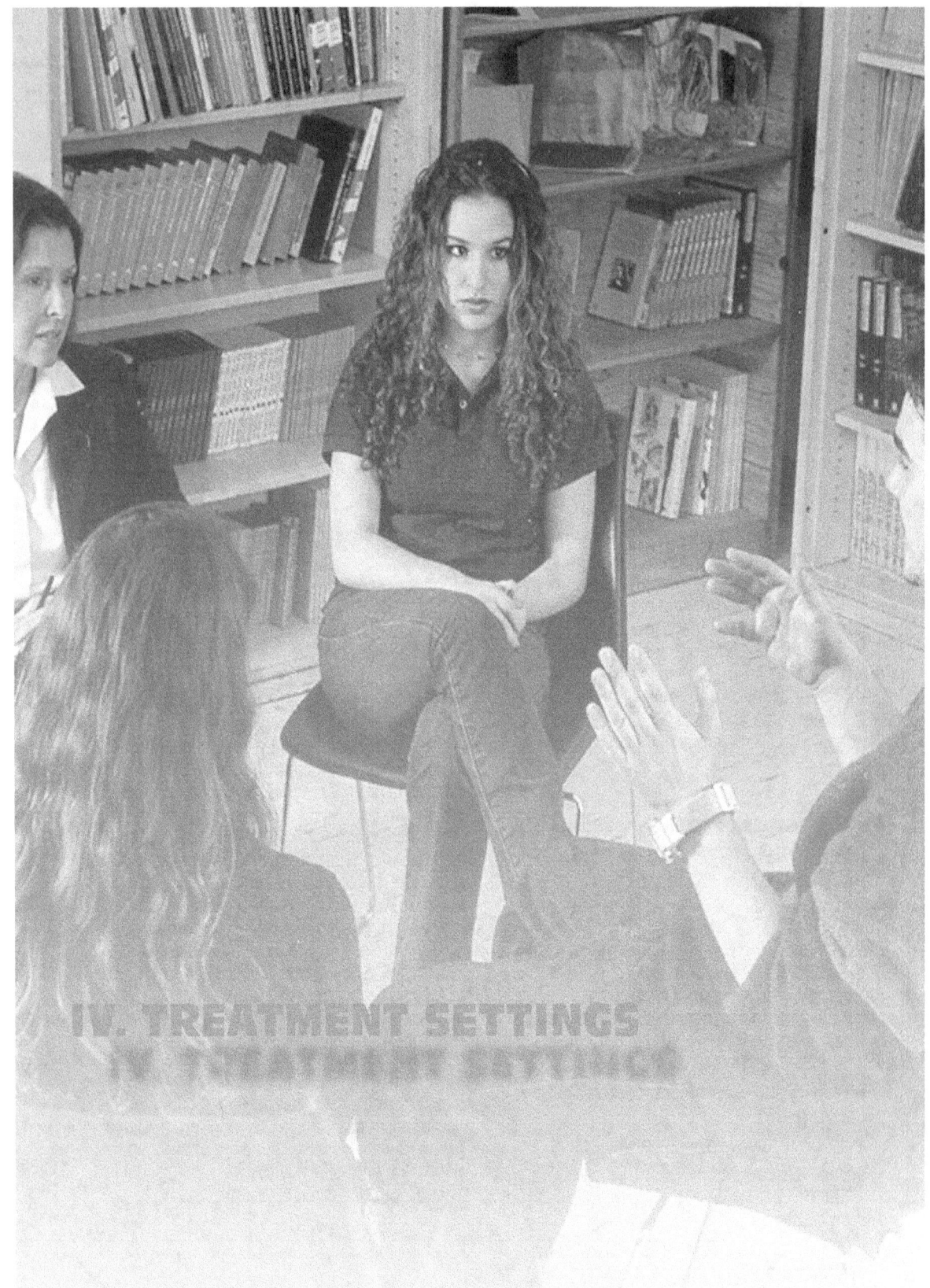

IV. TREATMENT SETTINGS

Treatment for substance use disorders is delivered at varying levels of care in many different settings. Because no single treatment is appropriate for every adolescent, treatments must be tailored for the individual. Based on the consensus of drug treatment experts, the American Society of Addiction Medicine (ASAM) has developed guidelines for determining the appropriate intensity and length of treatment for adolescents with substance abuse problems, based on an assessment involving six areas:[49]

(1) Level of intoxication and potential for withdrawal
(2) Presence of other medical conditions
(3) Presence of other emotional, behavioral, or cognitive conditions
(4) Readiness or motivation to change
(5) Risk of relapse or continued drug use
(6) Recovery environment (e.g., family, peers, school, legal system)

With a substance use disorder—as with any other medical condition—treatment must be long enough and strong enough to be effective. Just as an antibiotic must be taken for sufficient time to kill a bacterial infection, even though symptoms may already have subsided, substance abuse treatment must continue for a sufficient length of time to treat the disease. Undertreating a substance use disorder—providing lower than the recommended level of care or a shorter length of treatment than recommended—will increase the risk of relapse and could cause the patient, his or her family members, or the referring juvenile justice system to lose hope in the treatment because they will see it as ineffective.

This section will review the settings in which adolescent drug abuse treatment most often occurs.

Outpatient/Intensive Outpatient

Adolescent drug abuse treatment is most commonly offered in outpatient settings. When delivered by well-trained clinicians, this can be highly effective. Outpatient treatment is traditionally recommended for adolescents with less severe addictions, few additional mental health problems, and a supportive living environment, although evidence suggests that more severe cases can be treated in outpatient settings as well. Outpatient treatment varies in the type and intensity of services offered and may be delivered on an individual basis or in a group format (although research suggests group therapy can carry certain risks; see "Group Therapy for Adolescents," page 23). Low- or moderate-intensity outpatient care is generally delivered once or twice a week. Intensive outpatient services are delivered more frequently, typically more than twice a week for at least 3 hours per day. Outpatient programs may offer drug abuse prevention programming (focused on deterring further drug use) or other behavioral and family interventions.[50,51]

Partial Hospitalization

Adolescents with more severe substance use disorders but who can still be safely managed in their home living environment may be referred to a higher level of care called partial hospitalization or "day treatment." This setting offers adolescents the opportunity to participate in treatment 4–6 hours a day at least 5 days a week while living at home.[52]

Residential/Inpatient Treatment

Residential treatment is a resource-intense high level of care, generally for adolescents with severe levels of addiction whose mental health and medical needs and addictive behaviors require a 24-hour structured environment to make recovery possible. These adolescents may have complex psychiatric or medical problems or family issues that interfere with their ability to avoid substance use. One well-known long-term residential treatment model is the therapeutic community (TC). TCs use a combination of techniques to "resocialize" the adolescent and enlist all the members of the community, including residents and staff, as active participants in treatment. Treatment focuses on building personal and social responsibility and developing new coping skills. Such programs offer a range of family services and may require family participation if the TC is sufficiently close to where the family lives. Short-term residential programs also exist.[53]

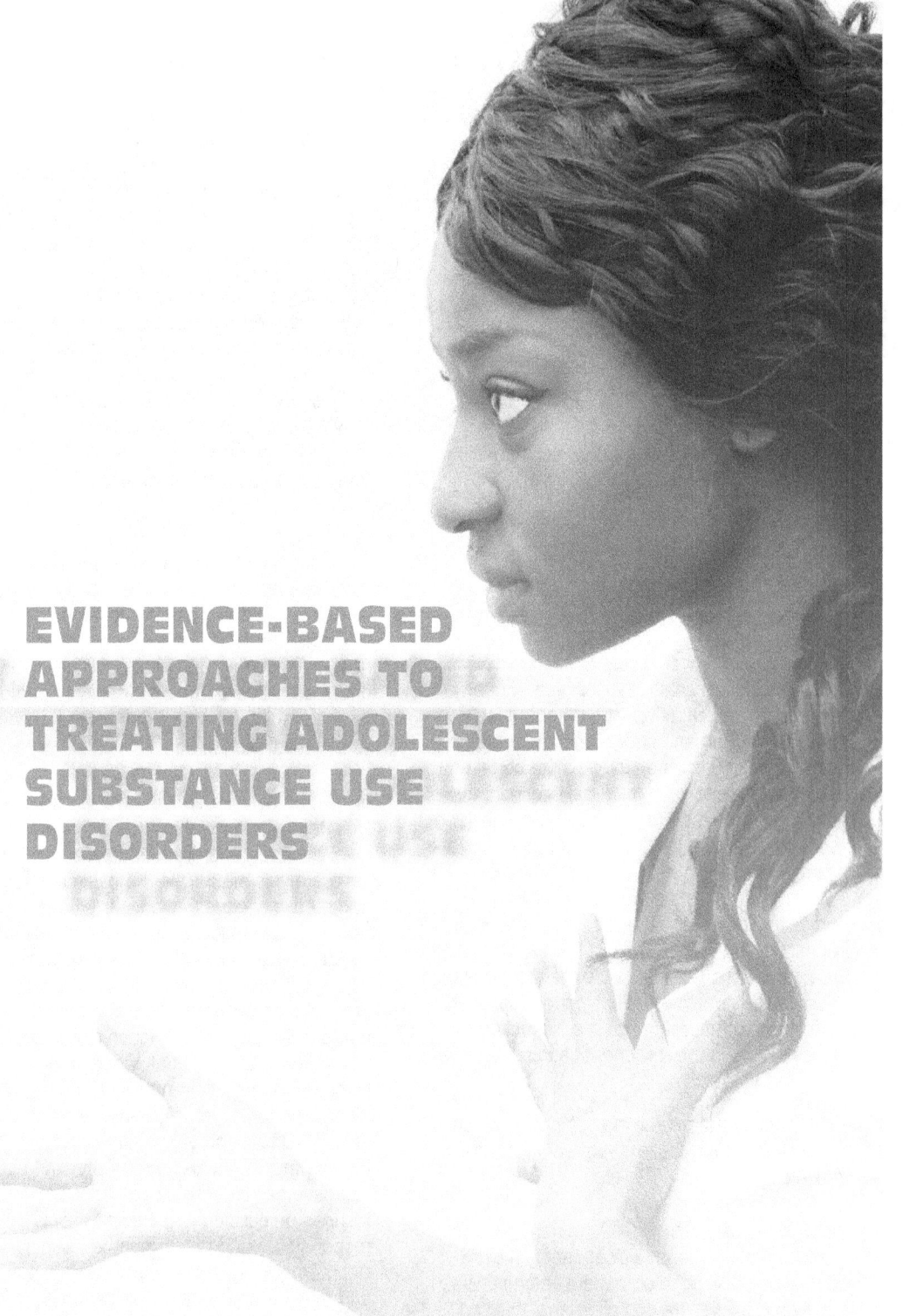

V. EVIDENCE-BASED APPROACHES TO TREATING ADOLESCENT SUBSTANCE USE DISORDERS

Research evidence supports the effectiveness of various substance abuse treatment approaches for adolescents. Examples of specific evidence-based approaches are described below, including behavioral and family-based interventions as well as medications. Each approach is designed to address specific aspects of adolescent drug use and its consequences for the individual, family, and society. In order for any intervention to be effective, the clinician providing it needs to be trained and well-supervised to ensure that he or she adheres to the instructions and guidance described in treatment manuals. Most of these treatments have been tested over short periods of 12–16 weeks, but for some adolescents, longer treatments may be warranted; such a decision is made on a case-by-case basis. The provider should use clinical judgment to select the evidence-based approach that seems best suited to the patient and his or her family.*

BEHAVIORAL APPROACHES

Behavioral interventions help adolescents to actively participate in their recovery from drug abuse and addiction and enhance their ability to resist drug use. In such approaches, therapists may provide incentives to remain abstinent, modify attitudes and behaviors related to drug abuse, assist families in improving their communication and overall interactions, and increase life skills to handle stressful circumstances and deal with environmental cues that may trigger intense craving for drugs. Below are some behavioral treatments shown to be effective in addressing substance abuse in adolescents (listed in alphabetical order).

Group Therapy for Adolescents

Adolescents can participate in group therapy and other peer support programs during and following treatment to help them achieve abstinence. When led by well-trained clinicians following well-validated Cognitive-Behavioral Therapy (CBT) protocols (see page 24), groups can provide positive social reinforcement through peer discussion and help enforce incentives to staying off drugs and living a drug-free lifestyle.

However, group treatment for adolescents carries a risk of unintended adverse effects: Group members may steer conversation toward talk that glorifies or extols drug use, thereby undermining recovery goals. Trained counselors need to be aware of that possibility and direct group activities and discussions in a positive direction.

Adolescent Community Reinforcement Approach (A-CRA)

A-CRA is an intervention that seeks to help adolescents achieve and maintain abstinence from drugs by replacing influences in their lives that had reinforced substance use with healthier family, social, and educational or vocational reinforcers. After assessing the adolescent's needs and levels of functioning, the therapist chooses from among 17 A-CRA procedures to address problem-solving, coping, and communication skills and to encourage active participation in constructive social and recreational activities.[54]

---

* The treatments listed in this book are not intended to be a comprehensive list of efficacious evidence-based treatment approaches for adolescents. NIDA continues supporting research developing new approaches to address adolescent drug abuse.

Cognitive-Behavioral Therapy (CBT)

CBT strategies are based on the theory that learning processes play a critical role in the development of problem behaviors like drug abuse. A core element of CBT is teaching participants how to anticipate problems and helping them develop effective coping strategies. In CBT, adolescents explore the positive and negative consequences of using drugs. They learn to monitor their feelings and thoughts and recognize distorted thinking patterns and cues that trigger their substance abuse; identify and anticipate high-risk situations; and apply an array of self-control skills, including emotional regulation and anger management, practical problem solving, and substance refusal. CBT may be offered in outpatient settings in either individual or group sessions (see "Group Therapy for Adolescents," page 23) or in residential settings.[55]

Contingency Management (CM)

Research has demonstrated the effectiveness of treatment using immediate and tangible reinforcements for positive behaviors to modify problem behaviors like substance abuse. This approach, known as Contingency Management (CM), provides adolescents an opportunity to earn low-cost incentives such as prizes or cash vouchers (for food items, movie passes, and other personal goods) in exchange for participating in drug treatment, achieving important goals of treatment, and not using drugs. The goal of CM is to weaken the influence of reinforcement derived from using drugs and to substitute it with reinforcement derived from healthier activities and drug abstinence. For adolescents, CM has been offered in a variety of settings, and parents can be trained to apply this method at home. CM is typically combined either with a psychosocial treatment or a medication (where available). Recent evidence also supports the use of Web-based CM to help adolescents stop smoking.[56]

Motivational Enhancement Therapy (MET)

MET is a counseling approach that helps adolescents resolve their ambivalence about engaging in treatment and quitting their drug use. This approach, which is based on a technique called motivational interviewing, typically includes an initial assessment of the adolescent's motivation to participate in treatment, followed by one to three individual sessions in which a therapist helps the patient develop a desire to participate in treatment by providing non-confrontational feedback. Being empathic yet directive, the therapist discusses the need for treatment and tries to elicit self-motivational statements from the adolescent to strengthen his or her motivation and build a plan for change. If the adolescent resists, the therapist responds neutrally rather than by contradicting or correcting the patient. MET, while better than no treatment, is typically not used as a stand-alone treatment for adolescents with substance use disorders but is used to motivate them to participate in other types of treatment.[57]

Twelve-Step Facilitation Therapy

Twelve-Step Facilitation Therapy is designed to increase the likelihood that an adolescent with a drug abuse problem will become affiliated and actively involved in a 12-step program like Alcoholics Anonymous (AA) or Narcotics Anonymous (NA). Such programs stress the participant's acceptance that life has become unmanageable, that abstinence from drug use is needed, and that willpower alone cannot overcome the problem. The benefits of 12-step participation for adults in extending the benefits of addiction treatment appear to apply to adolescent outpatients as well, according to recent research. Research also suggests adolescent-specific 12-step facilitation strategies may help enhance outpatient attendance rates.[58]

Behavioral interventions help adolescents to actively participate in their recovery from drug abuse and addiction and enhance their ability to resist drug use.

FAMILY-BASED APPROACHES

Family-based approaches to treating adolescent substance abuse highlight the need to engage the family, including parents, siblings, and sometimes peers, in the adolescent's treatment. Involving the family can be particularly important, as the adolescent will often be living with at least one parent and be subject to the parent's controls, rules, and/or supports. Family-based approaches generally address a wide array of problems in addition to the young person's substance problems, including family communication and conflict; other co-occurring behavioral, mental health, and learning disorders; problems with school or work attendance; and peer networks. Research shows that family-based treatments are highly efficacious; some studies even suggest they are superior to other individual and group treatment approaches.[59] Typically offered in outpatient settings, family treatments have also been tested successfully in higher-intensity settings such as residential and intensive outpatient programs. Below are specific types of family-based treatments shown to be effective in treating adolescent substance abuse.

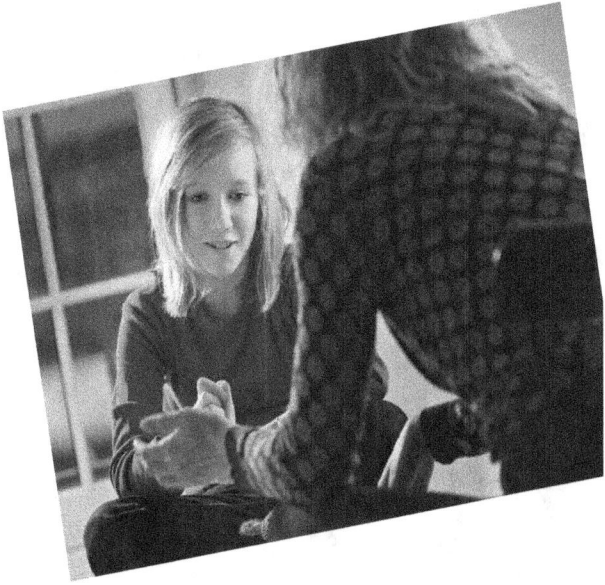

Brief Strategic Family Therapy (BSFT)

BSFT is based on a family systems approach to treatment, in which one member's problem behaviors are seen to stem from unhealthy family interactions. Over the course of 12–16 sessions, the BSFT counselor establishes a relationship with each family member, observes how the members behave with one another, and assists the family in changing negative interaction patterns. BSFT can be adapted to a broad range of family situations in various settings (mental health clinics, drug abuse treatment programs, social service settings, families' homes) and treatment modalities (as a primary outpatient intervention, in combination with residential or day treatment, or as an aftercare/continuing-care service following residential treatment).[60]

Family Behavior Therapy (FBT)

FBT, which has demonstrated positive results in both adults and adolescents, combines behavioral contracting with contingency management to address not only substance abuse but other behavioral problems as well. The adolescent and at least one parent participate in treatment planning and choose specific interventions from a menu of evidence-based treatment options. Therapists encourage family members to use behavioral strategies taught in sessions and apply their new skills to improve the home environment. They set behavioral goals for preventing substance use and reducing risk behaviors for sexually transmitted diseases like HIV, which are reinforced through a contingency management (CM) system (see description on page 24). Goals are reviewed and rewards provided at each session.[61]

Involving the family can be particularly important in adolescent substance abuse treatment.

Multidimensional Family Therapy (MDFT)

MDFT is a comprehensive family- and community-based treatment for substance-abusing adolescents and those at high risk for behavior problems such as conduct disorder and delinquency. The aim is to foster family competency and collaboration with other systems like school or juvenile justice. Sessions may take place in a variety of locations, including in the home, at a clinic, at school, at family court, or in other community locations. MDFT has been shown to be effective even with more severe substance use disorders and can facilitate the reintegration of substance abusing juvenile detainees into the community.[63]

Multisystemic Therapy (MST)

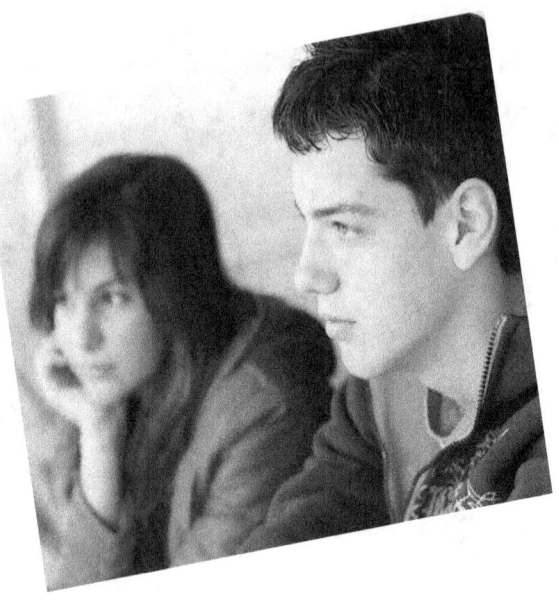

MST is a comprehensive and intensive family- and community-based treatment that has been shown to be effective even with adolescents whose substance abuse problems are severe and with those who engage in delinquent and/or violent behavior. In MST, the adolescent's substance abuse is viewed in terms of characteristics of the adolescent (e.g., favorable attitudes toward drug use) and those of his or her family (e.g., poor discipline, conflict, parental drug abuse), peers (e.g., positive attitudes toward drug use), school (e.g., dropout, poor performance), and neighborhood (e.g., criminal subculture). The therapist may work with the family as a whole but will also conduct sessions with just the caregivers or the adolescent alone.[64]

Functional Family Therapy (FFT)

FFT combines a family systems view of family functioning (which asserts that unhealthy family interactions underlie problem behaviors) with behavioral techniques to improve communication, problem-solving, conflict resolution, and parenting skills. Principal treatment strategies include (1) engaging families in the treatment process and enhancing their motivation for change and (2) modifying family members' behavior using CM techniques, communication and problem solving, behavioral contracts, and other methods.[62]

ADDICTION MEDICATIONS

Several medications have been found to be effective in treating addiction to opioids, alcohol, or nicotine in adults, although none of these medications have been approved by the FDA to treat adolescents. In most cases, only preliminary evidence exists for the effectiveness and safety of these medications in people under 18, and there is no evidence on the neurobiological impact of these medications

Undertreating a substance use disorder will increase the risk of relapse.

on the developing brain. However, despite the relative lack of evidence, some health care providers do use medications "off-label" when treating adolescents (especially older adolescents) who are addicted to opioids, nicotine, or (less commonly) alcohol. Newer compounds continue to be studied for possibly treating substance use disorders in adults and adolescents, but none other than those listed here have shown conclusive results.

Note that there are currently no FDA-approved medications to treat addiction to cannabis, cocaine, or methamphetamine in any age group.

Opioid Use Disorders

Buprenorphine reduces or eliminates opioid withdrawal symptoms, including drug cravings, without producing the "high" or dangerous side effects of heroin and other opioids. It does this by both activating and blocking opioid receptors in the brain (i.e., it is what is known as a partial opioid agonist). It is available for sublingual (under-the-tongue) administration both in a stand-alone formulation (called Subutex®) and in combination with another agent called naloxone. The naloxone in the combined formulation (marketed as Suboxone®) is included to deter diversion or abuse of the medication by causing a withdrawal reaction if it is intravenously injected.[65] Physicians with special certification may provide office-based buprenorphine treatment for detoxification and/or maintenance therapy.[66] It is sometimes prescribed to older adolescents on the basis of two research studies indicating its efficacy for this population,[67,68] even though it is not approved by the FDA for pediatric use.*

Methadone also prevents withdrawal symptoms and reduces craving in opioid-addicted individuals by activating opioid receptors in the brain (i.e., a full opioid agonist).

Adolescent drug abuse treatment is most commonly offered in outpatient settings.

It has a long history of use in treatment of opioid dependence in adults, and is available in specially licensed methadone treatment programs. In select cases and in some States, opioid-dependent adolescents between the ages of 16 and 18 may be eligible for methadone treatment, provided they have two documented failed treatments of opioid detoxification or drug-free treatment and have a written consent for methadone signed by a parent or legal guardian.[69]

Naltrexone is approved for the prevention of relapse in adult patients following complete detoxification from opioids. It acts by blocking the brain's opioid receptors (i.e., an opioid antagonist), preventing opioid drugs from acting on them and thus blocking the high the user would normally feel and/or causing withdrawal if recent opioid use has occurred. It can be taken orally in tablets or as a once-monthly injection given in a doctor's office (a preparation called Vivitrol®).[70]

Alcohol Use Disorders‡

Acamprosate (Campral®) reduces withdrawal symptoms by normalizing brain systems disrupted by chronic alcohol consumption in adults.

Disulfiram (Antabuse®) inhibits an enzyme involved in the metabolism of alcohol, causing an unpleasant reaction if alcohol is consumed after taking the medication.[71]

---

* According to the FDA label, "SUBOXONE and SUBUTEX are not recommended for use in pediatric patients. The safety and effectiveness of SUBOXONE and SUBUTEX in patients below the age of 16 have not been established."

‡ Medication-assisted therapies are rarely used to treat adolescent alcohol use disorders.

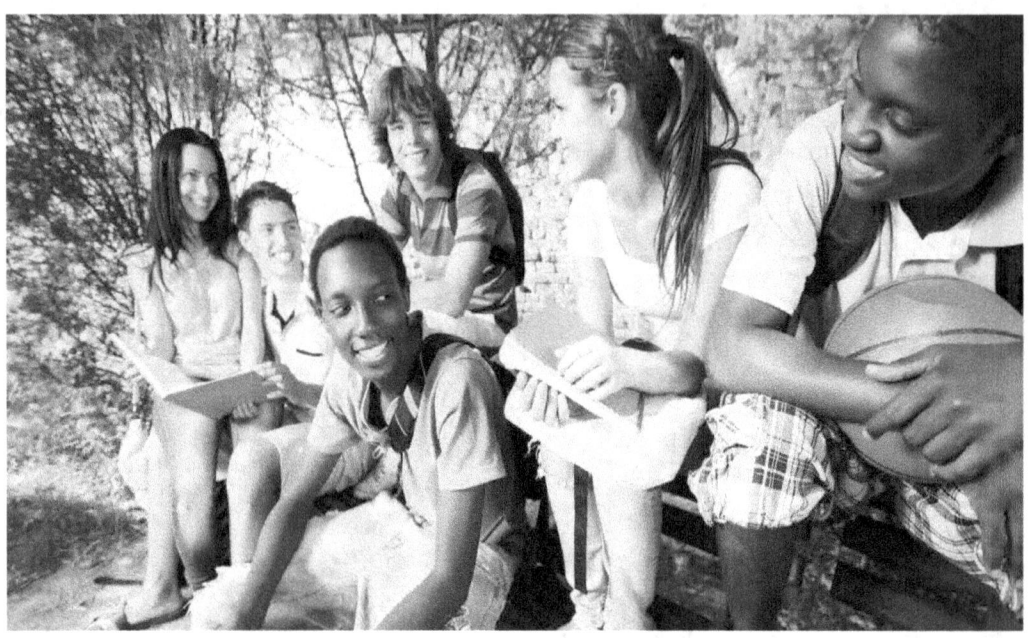

Naltrexone decreases alcohol-induced euphoria and is available in both oral tablets and long-acting injectable preparations (as in its use for the treatment of opioid addiction, above).

Nicotine Use Disorders

Bupropion, commonly prescribed for depression, also reduces nicotine cravings and withdrawal symptoms in adult smokers.[72]

Nicotine Replacement Therapies (NRTs) help smokers wean off cigarettes by activating nicotine receptors in the brain. They are available in the form of a patch, gum, lozenge, nasal spray, or inhaler.[73]

Varenicline reduces nicotine cravings and withdrawal in adult smokers by mildly stimulating nicotine receptors in the brain.[74]

RECOVERY SUPPORT SERVICES

To reinforce gains made in treatment and to improve their quality of life more generally, recovering adolescents may benefit from recovery support services, which include continuing care, mutual help groups (such as 12-step programs), peer recovery support services, and recovery high schools. Such programs provide a community setting where fellow recovering persons can share their experiences, provide mutual support to each other's struggles with drug or alcohol problems, and in other ways support a substance-free lifestyle. Note that recovery support services are not substitutes for treatment. Also, the existing research evidence for these approaches (with the exception of Assertive Continuing Care) is preliminary; anecdotal evidence supports the effectiveness of peer recovery support services and recovery high schools, for example, but their efficacy has not been established through controlled trials.

Assertive Continuing Care (ACC)

ACC is a home-based continuing-care approach delivered by trained clinicians to prevent relapse, and is typically used after an adolescent completes therapy utilizing the Adolescent Community Reinforcement Approach (A-CRA, see page 23). Using positive and negative reinforcement to shape behaviors, along with training in problem-solving and communication skills, ACC combines A-CRA and assertive case management services (e.g., use of a multidisciplinary team of professionals, round-the-clock coverage, assertive outreach) to help adolescents and their caregivers acquire the skills to engage in positive social activities.[75]

Mutual Help Groups

Mutual help groups such as the 12-step programs Alcoholics Anonymous (AA) and Narcotics Anonymous (NA) provide ongoing support for people with addictions to alcohol or drugs, respectively, free of charge and in a community setting. Participants meet in a group with others in recovery, once a week or more, sharing their experiences and offering mutual encouragement. Twelve-step groups are guided by a set of fundamental principles that participants are encouraged to adopt—including acknowledging that willpower alone cannot achieve sustained sobriety, that surrender to the group conscience must replace self-centeredness, and that long-term recovery involves a process of spiritual renewal.[76]

Peer Recovery Support Services

Peer recovery support services, such as recovery community centers, help individuals remain engaged in treatment and/or the recovery process by linking them together both in groups and in one-on-one relationships with peer leaders who have direct experience with addiction and recovery. Depending on the needs of the adolescent, peer leaders may provide mentorship and coaching and help connect individuals to treatment, 12-step groups, or other resources. Peer leaders may also facilitate or lead community-building activities, helping recovering adolescents build alternative social networks and have drug- and alcohol-free social options.[77]

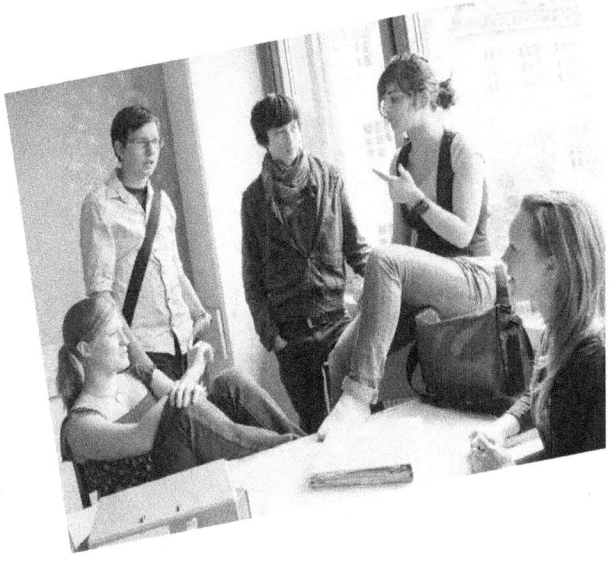

Recovery High Schools

Recovery high schools are schools specifically designed for students recovering from substance abuse issues. They are typically part of another school or set of alternative school programs within the public school system, but recovery school students are generally separated from other students by means of scheduling and physical barriers. Such programs allow adolescents newly in recovery to be surrounded by a peer group supportive of recovery efforts and attitudes. Recovery schools can serve as an adjunct to formal substance abuse treatment, with students often referred by treatment providers and enrolled in concurrent treatment for other mental health problems.[78]

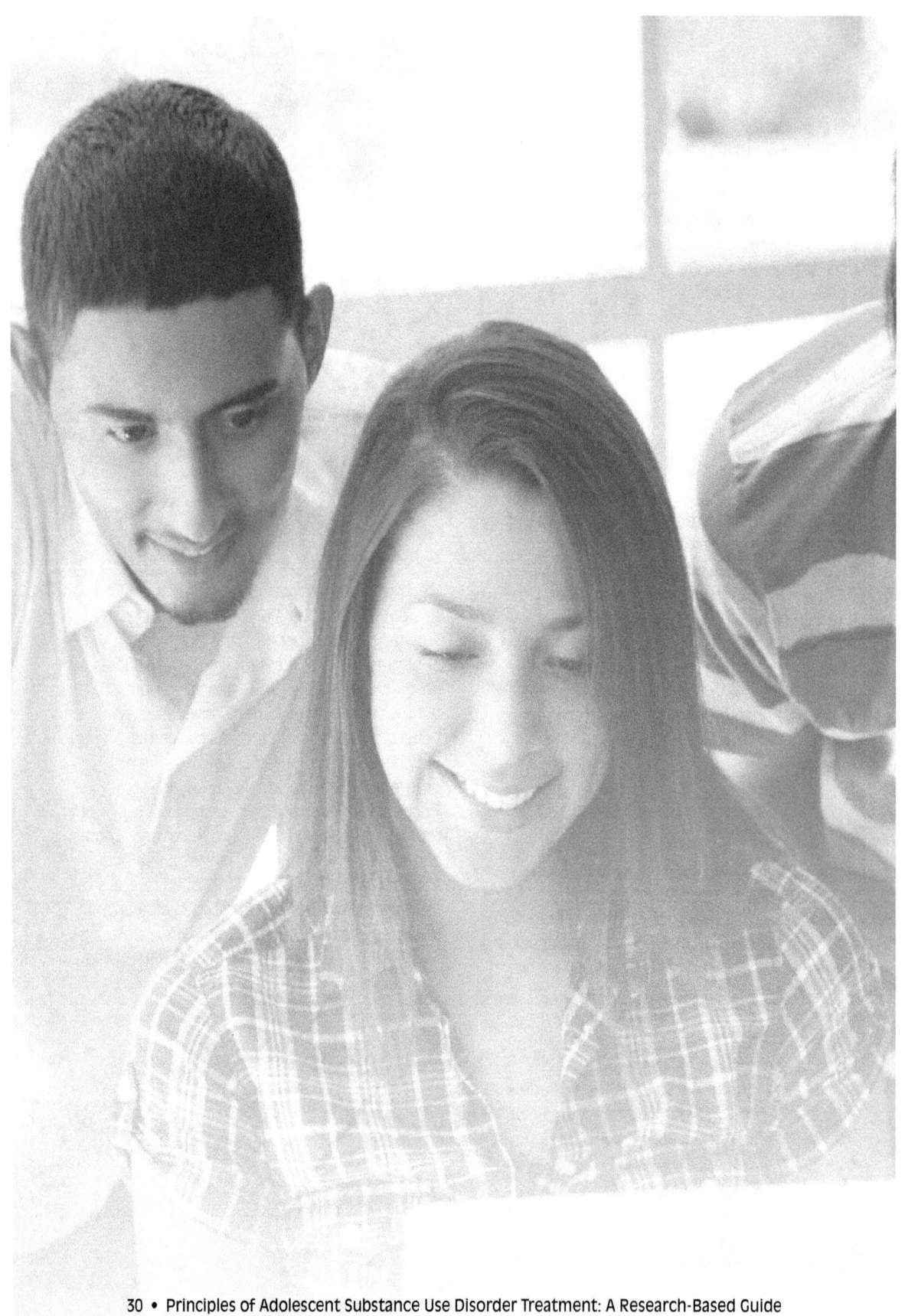

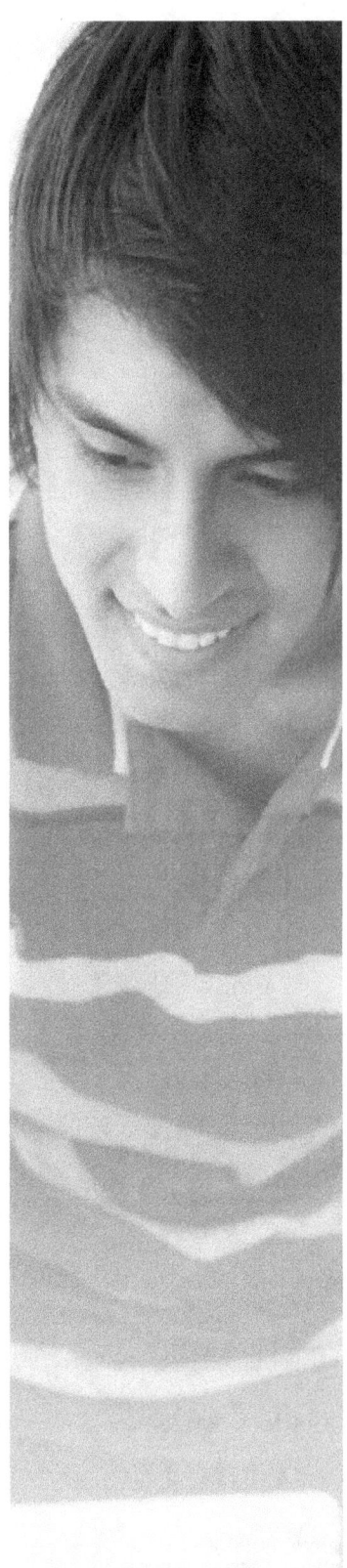

TREATMENT REFERRAL RESOURCES

Substance Abuse and Mental Health Services Administration (SAMHSA) Treatment Locator: 1-800-662-HELP or search www.findtreatment.samhsa.gov

The "Find A Physician" feature on the American Society of Addiction Medicine (ASAM) Web site:
http://community.asam.org/search/default.asp?m=basic

The Patient Referral Program on the American Academy of Addiction Psychiatry Web site:
http://www.aaap.org/patient-referral-program

The Child and Adolescent Psychiatrist Finder on the American Academy of Child and Adolescent Psychiatry Web site:
http://www.aacap.org/cs/root/child_and_adolescent_psychiatrist_finder/child_and_adolescent_psychiatrist_finder

References

1. Johnston, L.D.; O'Malley, P.M.; Bachman, J.G.; and Schulenberg, J.E. *Monitoring the Future National Results on Adolescent Drug Use: Overview of Key Findings, 2013.* Bethesda, MD: National Institute on Drug Abuse, 2013. Available at www.monitoringthefuture.org

2. Sussman, S.; Skara, S.; and Ames, S.L. Substance abuse among adolescents. *Substance Use & Misuse* 43(12–13):1802–1828, 2008.

3. Robertson, E.B.; David, S.L.; and Rao, S.A. *Preventing Drug Use among Children and Adolescents: A Research-Based Guide for Parents, Educators, and Community Leaders,* 2nd ed. NIH Pub. No. 04-4212(A). Bethesda, MD: National Institute on Drug Abuse, 2003. Available at: http://www.drugabuse.gov/pdf/prevention/RedBook.pdf

4. Andersen, S.L.; and Teicher, M.H. Desperately driven and no brakes: Developmental stress exposure and subsequent risk for substance abuse. *Neuroscience & Biobehavioral Reviews* 33(4):516–524, 2009.

5. Andersen, S.L.; and Teicher, M.H. Desperately driven and no brakes: Developmental stress exposure and subsequent risk for substance abuse. *Neuroscience & Biobehavioral Reviews* 33(4):516–524, 2009.

6. Robertson, E.B.; David, S.L.; and Rao, S.A. *Preventing Drug Use among Children and Adolescents: A Research-Based Guide for Parents, Educators, and Community Leaders,* 2nd ed. NIH Pub. No. 04-4212(A). Bethesda, MD: National Institute on Drug Abuse, 2003. Available at: http://www.drugabuse.gov/pdf/prevention/RedBook.pdf

7. Dennis, M.; Babor, T.F.; Roebuck, C.; and Donaldson, J. Changing the focus: The case for recognizing and treating cannabis use disorders. *Addiction* 97:(s1):4–15, 2002.

8. Substance Abuse and Mental Health Services Administration. *Results from the 2012 National Survey on Drug Use and Health: Summary of National Findings.* NSDUH Series H-46, HHS Publication No. (SMA) 13-4795. Rockville, MD: Substance Abuse and Mental Health Services Administration, 2013.

9. McCabe, S.E.; West, B.T.; Morales, M.; Cranford, J.A.; and Boyd, C.J. Does early onset of non-medical use of prescription drugs predict subsequent prescription drug abuse and dependence? Results from a national study. *Addiction* 102(12):1920–1930, 2007.

10. Substance Abuse and Mental Health Services Administration. *Results from the 2012 National Survey on Drug Use and Health: Summary of National Findings.* NSDUH Series H-46, HHS Publication No. (SMA) 13-4795. Rockville, MD: Substance Abuse and Mental Health Services Administration, 2013.

11. Meier, M.H.; Caspi, A.; Ambler, A.; Harrington, H.L.; Houts, R.; Keefe, R.S.E.; McDonald, K.; Ward, A.; Poulton, R.; and Moffitt, T.E. Persistent cannabis users show neuropsychological decline from childhood to midlife *Proceedings of the National Academy of Sciences of the United States of America* Oct 2;109(40):E2657–E2664, 2012.

12. Dennis, M.L.; White, M.; and Ives, M.I. Individual characteristics and needs associated with substance misuse of adolescents and young adults in addiction treatment. In Carl Leukefeld, Tom Gullotta, and Michele Staton Tindall (eds.), *Handbook on Adolescent Substance Abuse Prevention and Treatment: Evidence-Based Practice.* New London, CT: Child and Family Agency Press, 2009.

13. Chan, Y.F.; Godley, M.D.; Godley, S.H.; and Dennis, M.L. Utilization of mental health services among adolescents in community-based substance abuse outpatient clinics. *The Journal of Behavioral Health Services & Research*, Special Issue 35(1):35–51, 2009.

14. Office of Applied Studies, Substance Abuse and Mental Health Services Administration. Quantity and frequency of alcohol use among underage drinkers. *The NSDUH Report*: March 31, 2008. Available at: http://www.samhsa.gov/data/2k8/underage/underage.htm

15. Breda, C.; and Heflinger, C.A. Predicting incentives to change among adolescents with substance abuse disorder. *The American Journal of Drug and Alcohol Abuse* 30(2):251–267, 2004.

16. Substance Abuse and Mental Health Services Administration. *Results from the 2012 National Survey on Drug Use and Health: Summary of National Findings.* NSDUH Series H-46, HHS Publication No. (SMA) 13-4795. Rockville, MD: Substance Abuse and Mental Health Services Administration, 2013.

17. National Institute on Drug Abuse. *Drugs, Brains, and Behavior: The Science of Addiction.* NIH Pub. No. 10-5605, Revised August 2010. Available at: http://www.drugabuse.gov/publications/science-addiction

18. American Society of Addiction Medicine. *ASAM Patient Placement Criteria for the Treatment of Substance Related Disorders,* 2nd Edition. Chevy Chase, MD: American Society of Addiction Medicine, 2001.

19. Committee on Substance Abuse, American Academy of Pediatrics. Substance use screening, brief intervention, and referral to treatment for pediatricians. *Pediatrics* 128;e1330; 2011. Available at: http://pediatrics.aappublications.org/content/early/2011/10/26/peds.2011-1754.full.pdf

20. National Institute on Alcohol Abuse and Alcoholism. *Alcohol screening and brief intervention for youth: A practitioner's guide*. NIH Pub. No. 11-7805, 2011. Available at: http://pubs.niaaa.nih.gov/publications/Practitioner/YouthGuide/YouthGuide.pdf

21. Committee on Substance Abuse, American Academy of Pediatrics. Substance use screening, brief intervention, and referral to treatment for pediatricians. *Pediatrics* 128;e1330, 2011. Available at: http://pediatrics.aappublications.org/content/early/2011/10/26/peds.2011-1754.full.pdf

22. Miller, N.S.; and Flaherty, J.A. Effectiveness of coerced addiction treatment (alternative consequences): A review of the clinical research. *Journal of Substance Abuse Treatment* 18(1):9–16, 2000.

23. Chan, Y.F.; Dennis, M.L.; and Funk, R.R. Prevalence and comorbidity co-occurrence of major internalizing and externalizing disorders among adolescents and adults presenting to substance abuse treatment. *Journal of Substance Abuse Treatment* 34:14–24, 2008

24. Simpson, T.L.; and Miller, W.R. Concomitance between childhood sexual and physical abuse and substance use problems: A review. *Clinical Psychology Review* 22(1):27–77, 2002.

25. Hser, Y.; Grella, C.E.; Hubbard, R.L.; Hsieh, S.C.; Fletcher, B.W.; Brown, B.S.; and Anglin, M.D. An evaluation of drug treatments for adolescents in 4 US cities. *Archives of General Psychiatry* 58(7):689–695, 2001.

26. Godley, M.D.; Godley, S.H.; Dennis, M.L.; Funk, R.R.; and Passetti, L.L. The effect of continuing care on continuing care linkage, adherence and abstinence following residential treatment for adolescents with substance use disorders. *Addiction* 102(1), 2006.

27. Godley, M.D.; Godley, S.H.; Dennis, M.L.; Funk, R.R.; and Passetti, L.L. The effect of assertive continuing care on continuing care linkage, adherence and abstinence following residential treatment for adolescents with substance use disorders. *Addiction* 102(1):81–93, 2007.

28. Lambert, E.Y.; Normand, JL.; and Volkow, N.D. Prevention and treatment of HIV/AIDS among drug-using populations: A global perspective. *Journal of Acquired Immune Deficiency Syndromes* 55(Suppl 1):S1–S4, 2010.

29. Hagan, H.; Pouget, E.R.; and Des Jarlais, D.C. A systematic review and meta-analysis of interventions to prevent hepatitis C virus infection in people who inject drugs. *Journal of Infectious Diseases* 204(1):74–83, 2011.

30. Shane, P.; Diamond, G.S.; Mensinger, J.L.; Shera, D.; and Wintersteen, M.B. Impact of victimization on substance abuse treatment outcomes for adolescents in outpatient and residential substance abuse treatment. *The American Journal on Addictions* 15, Issue Supplement s1:s34–s42, 2010.

31. Nash, S.G.; McQueen, A.; and Bray, J.H. Pathways to adolescent alcohol use: Family environment, peer influence, and parental expectations. *Journal of Adolescent Health* 37(1):19–28, 2005.

32. Hall, W.; and Degenhardt, L. Adverse health effects of non-medical cannabis use. *Lancet* 374:1383–1391, 2009.

33. Johnston, L.D.; O'Malley, P.M.; Bachman, J.G.; and Schulenberg, J.E. *Monitoring the Future National Results on Adolescent Drug Use: Overview of Key Findings, 2013*. Bethesda, MD: National Institute on Drug Abuse, 2013. Available at www.monitoringthefuture.org

34. Storra, C.L.; Westergaard, R.; and Anthony, J.C. Early onset inhalant use and risk for opiate initiation by young adulthood. *Drug and Alcohol Dependence* 78(3): 253–261, 2005

35. Pollini, R.A.; Banta-Green, C.J.; Cuevas-Mota, J.; Metzner, M.; Teshale, E.; and Garfein, R.S. Problematic use of prescription-type opioids prior to heroin use among young heroin injectors. *Substance Abuse and Rehabilitation* 2:173–180, 2011.

36. Ilieva, I.; Boland, J.; and Farah, M.J. Objective and subjective cognitive enhancing effects of mixed amphetamine salts in healthy people. *Neuropharmacology* 64:496–505, 2013.

37. Kanayama, G.; Brower, K.J.; Wood, R.I.; Hudson, J.I.; and Pope, H.G., Jr. Treatment of anabolic-androgenic steroid dependence: Emerging evidence and its implications. *Drug and Alcohol Dependence* 109(1-3): 6–13, 2010.

38. Skarberg, K.; Nyberg, F.; and Engstrom, I. Multisubstance use as a feature of addiction to anabolic-androgenic steroids. *European Addiction Research* 15(2):99–106, 2009.

39. Humphreys K.L.; Eng, T; and Lee, S.S. Stimulant medication and substance use outcomes: A meta-analysis. *JAMA Psychiatry* 1–9, 2013.

40. Committee on Substance Abuse, American Academy of Pediatrics. Substance use screening, brief intervention, and referral to treatment for pediatricians. *Pediatrics* 128(5):e1330–1340, 2011. Available at: http://pediatrics.aappublications.org/content/early/2011/10/26/peds.2011-1754.full.pdf

41. Kulig, J.W.; and the Committee on Substance Abuse, American Academy of Pediatrics. Tobacco, alcohol, and other drugs: The role of the pediatrician in prevention, identification, and management of substance abuse. *Pediatrics* 115(3):816–821, 2005.

42. Committee on Substance Abuse, American Academy of Pediatrics. Substance use screening, brief intervention, and referral to treatment for pediatricians. *Pediatrics* 128(5):e1330–1340, 2011. Available at: http://pediatrics.aappublications.org/content/early/2011/10/26/peds.2011-1754.full.pdf

43. National Institute on Alcohol Abuse and Alcoholism. *Alcohol screening and brief intervention for youth: A practitioner's guide*. NIH Pub. No. 11-7805, 2011. Available at: http://pubs.niaaa.nih.gov/publications/Practitioner/YouthGuide/YouthGuide.pdf

44. Rosen I.M.; and Maurer, D.M. Reducing tobacco use in adolescents. *American Family Physician* 77(4):483–490, 2008.

45. Substance Abuse and Mental Health Services Administration. *Results from the 2012 National Survey on Drug Use and Health: Summary of National Findings*. NSDUH Series H-46, HHS Publication No. (SMA) 13-4795. Rockville, MD: Substance Abuse and Mental Health Services Administration, 2013.

46. Henggeler, S.W.; Halliday-Boykins, C.A.; Cunningham, P.B.; Randall, J.; Shapiro, S.B.; and Chapman, J.E. Juvenile drug court: Enhancing outcomes by integrating evidence-based treatments. *Journal of Consulting and Clinical Psychology* 74(1):42–54, 2006.

47. Ives, M.L.; Chan, Y.; Modisette, K.C.; and Dennis, M.L. Characteristics, needs, services and outcomes of youth in Juvenile Drug Courts (JTDC) compared to adolescent outpatient (AOP). *Drug Court Review*, 7(1):10–56, 2010.

48. McClelland, G.M.; Teplin, L.A.; and Abram, K.M. Detection and prevalence of substance use among juvenile detainees. *Juvenile Justice Bulletin*. Washington, DC: U.S. Department of Justice, Office of Justice Programs, Office of Juvenile Justice and Delinquency Prevention, 2004.

49. American Society of Addiction Medicine. *ASAM Patient Placement Criteria for the Treatment of Substance Related Disorders*, 2nd Edition. Chevy Chase, MD: American Society of Addiction Medicine, 2001.

50. Balsa, A.I.; Homer, J.F.; French, M.T.; and Weisner, C.M. Substance use, education, employment, and criminal activity outcomes of adolescents in outpatient chemical dependency programs. *Journal of Behavioral Health Services and Research* Jan;36(1):75–95, 2009.

51. Tanner-Smith, E.E.; Wilson, S.J.; and Lipsey, M.W. The comparative effectiveness of outpatient treatment for adolescent substance abuse: A meta-analysis. *Journal of Substance Abuse Treatment* 44(2):145–158, 2013.

52. Liddle, H.A.; Rowe, C.L.; Gonzalez, A.;; Henderson, C.E.; Dakof, G.A.; and Greenbaum, P.E. Changing provider practices, program environment, and improving outcomes by transporting multidimensional family therapy to an adolescent drug treatment setting. *American Journal on Addictions* 15:Suppl 1:102–112, 2006.

53. Morral, A.R.; McCaffrey, D.F.; and Ridgeway, G. Effectiveness of community-based treatment for substance-abusing adolescents: 12-month outcomes of youths entering Phoenix Academy or alternative probation dispositions. *Psychology of Addictive Behaviors* Sep;18(3):257–268, 2004.

54. Dennis, M.; Godley, S.H.; Diamond, G.; Tims, F.M.; Babor, T.; Donaldson, J.; Liddle, H.; Titus, J.C.; Kaminer, Y.; Webb, C.; Hamilton, N.; and Funk, R. The Cannabis Youth Treatment (CYT) Study: Main findings from two randomized trials. *Journal of Substance Abuse Treatment* 27(3):197–213, 2004.

55. Kaminer, Y.; and Waldron, H.B. Evidence-based cognitive behavioral therapies for adolescent substance use disorders: Applications and challenges. In C. Rowe & H. Liddle (eds.), *Adolescent substance abuse: Research and clinical advances*. New York: Cambridge University Press, pp. 396–419, 2006.

56. Stanger, C.; and Budney, A.J.; Contingency management approaches for adolescent substance use disorders. *Child and Adolescent Psychiatric Clinics of North America* 19(3):547–562, 2010.

57. Barnett, E.; Sussman, S.; Smith, C.; Rohrbach, L.A.; and Spruijt-Metz, D. Motivational Interviewing for adolescent substance use: a review of the literature. *Addictive Behaviors* 37(12):1325–1334, 2012.

58. Kelly, J.F.; and Urbanoski, K. Youth recovery contexts: The incremental effects of 12-step attendance and involvement on adolescent outpatient outcomes. *Alcoholism, Clinical and Experimental Research* 36(7):1219–1229, 2012.

59. Hogue, A.; and Liddle, H.A. Family-based treatment for adolescent substance abuse: controlled trials and new horizons in services research. *Journal of Family Therapy* 31(2):126–154, 2009.

60. Robbins, M.S.; Feaster, D.J.; Horigian, V.E.; Rohrbaugh, M.; Shoham, V.; Bachrach, K.;; Miller, M., Burlew, K.A.; Hodgkins, C.; Carrion, I.; Vandermark, N.; Schindler, E.; Werstlein, R.; and Szapocznik, J. Brief strategic family therapy versus treatment as usual: Results of a multisite randomized trial for substance using adolescents. *Journal of Consulting and Clinical Psychology* 79(6):713–727, 2011.

61. Donohue, B., Allen, D.A., and Lapota, H. Family Behavior Therapy. In D. Springer; and A. Rubin (eds.), *Substance Abuse Treatment for Youth and Adults*. New York: John Wiley & Sons, Inc., pp. 205–255, 2009.

62. Waldron, H.B.; Turner, C.W.; and Ozechowski, T.J. Profiles of drug use behavior change for adolescents in treatment. *Addictive Behaviors* 30(9):1775–1796, 2005.

63. Liddle, H.A.; Dakof, G.A.; Henderson, C.; and Rowe, C. Implementation outcomes of multidimensional family therapy-detention to community: A reintegration program for drug-using juvenile detainees. *International Journal of Offender Therapy and Comparative Criminology* 55(4):587–604, 2011.

64. Sheidow, A.J.; and Henggeler, S.W. Multisystemic therapy with substance using adolescents: A synthesis of the research. In N. Jainchill (Ed.), *Understanding and Treating Adolescent Substance use Disorders: Assessment, Treatment, Juvenile Justice Responses*. Kingston, NJ: Civic Research Institute, pp. 9-1–9-22, 2012.

65. Subramaniam, G.A.; Warden, D.; Minhajuddin, A.; Fishman, M.J.; Stitzer, M.L.; Adinoff, B.; Trivedi, M.; Weiss, R.; Potter, J.; Poole, S.A.; and Woody, G.E. Predictors of abstinence: National Institute on Drug Abuse multisite buprenorphine/naloxone treatment trial in opioid-dependent youth. *Journal of the American Academy of Child and Adolescent Psychiatry* 50(11):1120–1128, 2011.

66. Substance Abuse and Mental Health Services Administration. Physician Waiver Qualifications. Available at: http://buprenorphine.samhsa.gov/waiver_qualifications.html

67. Woody, G.E.; Poole, S.A.; Subramaniam, G.; Dugosh, K.; Bogenschutz, M.; Abbott, P.; Patkar, A.; Publicker, M.; McCain, K.; Potter, J.S.; Forman, R.; Vetter, V.;, McNicholas, L.; Blaine, J.; Lynch, K.G.; and Fudala, P. Extended vs short-term buprenorphine-naloxone for treatment of opioid-addicted youth: a randomized trial. *Journal of the American Medical Association* 300(17):2003–2011, 2008. Erratum in *Journal of the American Medical Association* 301(8):830, 2009.

68. Marsch, L.A.; Bickel, W.K.; Badger, G.J.; Stothart, M.E.; Quesnel, K.J.; Stanger, C.; and Brooklyn, J. Comparison of pharmacological treatments for opioid-dependent adolescents: A randomized controlled trial. *Archives of General Psychiatry* 62(10):1157–1164, 2005.

69. Marsch, L.A. Treatment of adolescents. In Strain, E.C.; and Stitzer, M.L. (eds.) *The Treatment of Opioid Dependence*. Baltimore, MD: Johns Hopkins University Press, pp. 497–507, 2005.

70. Fishman, M.J.; Winstanley, E.L.; Curran, E.; Garrett, S.; and Subramaniam, G. Treatment of opioid dependence in adolescents and young adults with extended release naltrexone: Preliminary case-series and feasibility. *Addiction* 105(9):1669–1676, 2010.

71. Niederhofer, H.; and Staffen, W. Comparison of disulfiram and placebo in treatment of alcohol dependence of adolescents. *Drug and Alcohol Review* 22(3):295–297, 2003.

72. Gray, K.M.; Carpenter, M.J.; Baker, N.L.; Hartwell, K.J.; Lewis, A.L.; Hiott, D.W.; Deas, D.; and Upadhyaya, H.P. Bupropion SR and contingency management for adolescent smoking cessation. *Journal of Substance Abuse Treatment* 40(1):77–86, 2011.

73. Moolchan, E.T.; Robinson, M.L.; Ernst, M.; Cadet, J.L.; Pickworth, W.B.; Heishman, S.J.; and Schroeder, J.R. Safety and efficacy of the nicotine patch and gum for the treatment of adolescent tobacco addiction. *Pediatrics* 115(4):e407–414, 2005.

74. Gray, K.M.; Carpenter, M.J.; Lewis, A.L.; Klintworth, E.M.; and Upadhyaya, H.P. Varenicline versus bupropion XL for smoking cessation in older adolescents: A randomized, double-blind pilot trial. *Nicotine and Tobacco Research* 14(2):234–239, 2012.

75. Godley, M.D.; Godley, S.H.; Dennis, M.L.; Funk, R.R.; and Passetti, L.L. The effect of assertive continuing care on continuing care linkage, adherence and abstinence following residential treatment for adolescents with substance use disorders. *Addiction* 102(1):81–93, 2007.

76. Kelly, J.F.; Dow, S.J.; Yeterian, J.D.; and Kahler, C.W. Can 12-step group participation strengthen and extend the benefits of adolescent addiction treatment? A prospective analysis. *Drug and Alcohol Dependence*, 110(1-2):117–125, 2010.

77. Substance Abuse and Mental Health Services Administration. *What are peer recovery support services?* Rockville, MD: Substance Abuse and Mental Health Services Administration, 2009. Available at: http://store.samhsa.gov/shin/content/SMA09-4454/SMA09-4454.pdf

78. Moberg, D.P.; and Finch, A.J. Recovery high schools: A descriptive study of school programs and students. *Journal of Groups in Addiction & Recovery* 2:128–161, 2008.

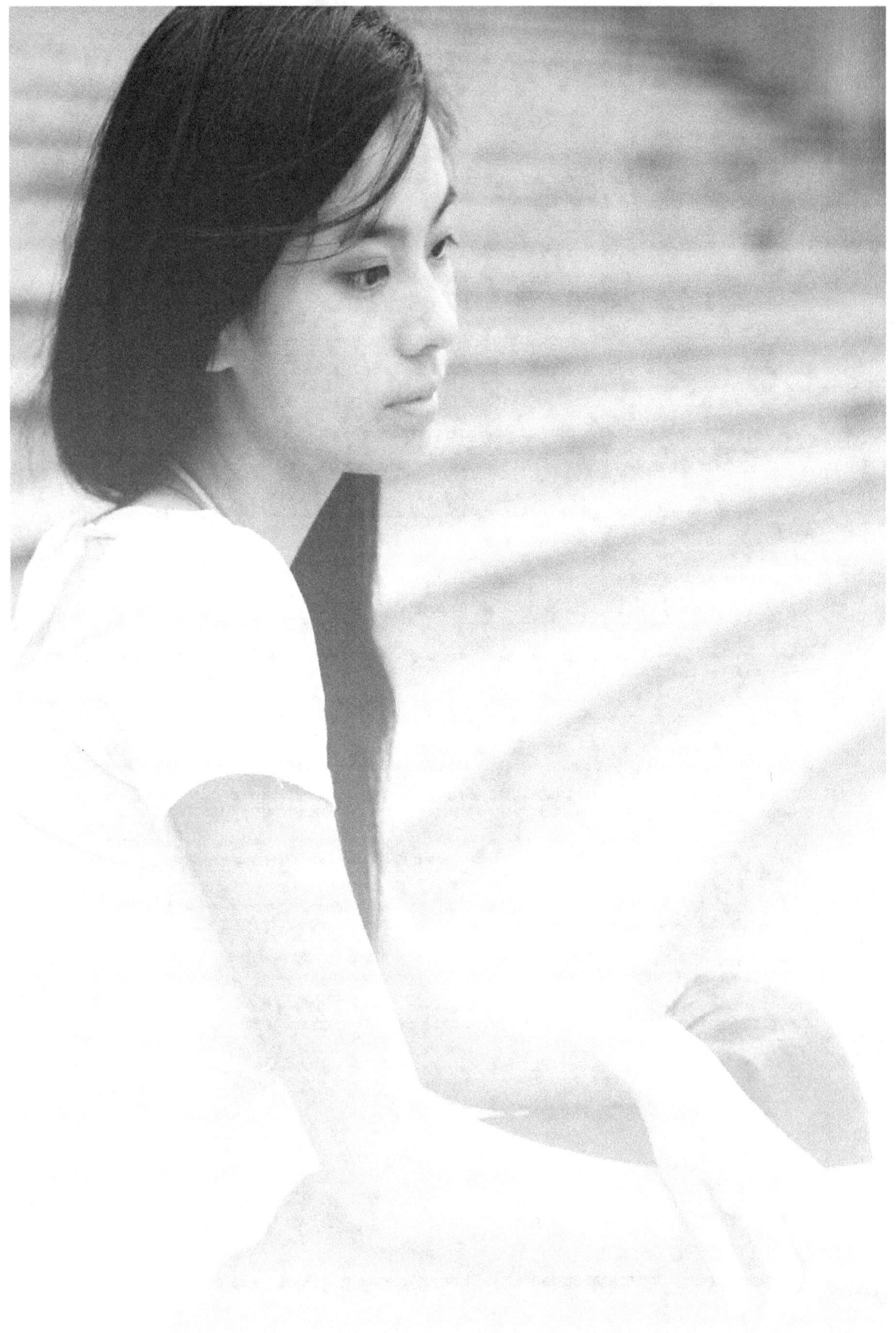

www.ingramcontent.com/pod-product-compliance
Lightning Source LLC
Chambersburg PA
CBHW082123220526
45472CB00009B/2281